Oncology imaging: Updates and Advancements

Editor

NATALIE S. LUI

SURGICAL ONCOLOGY CLINICS OF NORTH AMERICA

www.surgonc.theclinics.com

Consulting Editor
TIMOTHY M. PAWLIK

October 2022 • Volume 31 • Number 4

ELSEVIER

1600 John F. Kennedy Boulevard • Suite 1800 • Philadelphia, Pennsylvania, 19103-2899

http://www.theclinics.com

SURGICAL ONCOLOGY CLINICS OF NORTH AMERICA Volume 31, Number 4
October 2022 ISSN 1055-3207, ISBN-13: 978-0-323-98791-2

Editor: John Vassallo (j.vassallo@elsevier.com)
Developmental Editor: Diana Ang

Surgical Oncology Clinics of North America (ISSN 1055-3207) is published quarterly by Elsevier Inc., 360 Park Avenue South, New York, NY 10010-1710. Months of publication are January, April, July, and October. Business and Editorial Offices: 1600 John F. Kennedy Blvd., Ste. 1800, Philadelphia, PA 19103-2899. Customer Service Office: 3251 Riverport Lane, Maryland Heights, MO 63043. Periodicals postage paid at New York, NY and additional mailing offices. Subscription prices are $325.00 per year (US individuals), $776.00 (US institutions) $100.00 (US student/resident), $363.00 (Canadian individuals), $803.00 (Canadian institutions), $100.00 (Canadian student/resident), $470.00 (foreign individuals), $803.00 (foreign institutions), and $205.00 (foreign student/resident). Foreign air speed delivery is included in all *Clinics* subscription prices. All prices are subject to change without notice. **POSTMASTER**: Send address changes to *Surgical Oncology Clinics of North America,* Elsevier Health Science Division, Subscription Customer Service, 3251 Riverport Lane, Maryland Heights, MO 63043. **Customer Service: 1-800-654-2452 (US and Canada). 314-447-8871 (outside US and Canada). Fax: 314-447-8029. E-mail: journalscustomerservice-usa@elsevier.com (for print support); journalsonline support-usa@elsevier.com (for online support).**

Reprints. For copies of 100 or more, of articles in this publication, please contact the Commercial Reprints Department, Elsevier Inc., 360 Park Avenue South, New York, New York 10010-1710. Tel. 212-633-3874; Fax: 212-633-3820; E-mail: reprints@elsevier.com.

Surgical Oncology Clinics of North America is covered in *MEDLINE/PubMed (Index Medicus)* and *EMBASE/ Excerpta Medica, Current Contents/Clinical Medicine, and ISI/BIOMED.*

Contributors

CONSULTING EDITOR

TIMOTHY M. PAWLIK, MD, PhD, MPH, MTS, MBA, FACS, FSSO, FRACS (Hon.)
Professor and Chair, Department of Surgery, The Urban Meyer III and Shelley Meyer Chair for Cancer Research, Professor of Surgery, Oncology, Health Services Management and Policy, The Ohio State University, Wexner Medical Center, Columbus, Ohio, USA

EDITOR

NATALIE S. LUI, MD, MAS
Assistant Professor of Cardiothoracic Surgery, Stanford School of Medicine, Stanford, California, USA

AUTHORS

MARY KATHRYN ABEL, AB
School of Medicine, University of California, San Francisco, San Francisco, California, USA

CATHERINE T. BYRD, MD
Postdoctoral fellow, Department of Cardiothoracic Surgery, Stanford University, Stanford, California, USA

GLORIA Y. CHANG, MD
Department of Surgery, Division of Surgical Oncology, University of Texas Southwestern Medical Center, Dallas, Texas, USA

QUAN-YANG DUH, MD
Chief, Section of Endocrine Surgery, Professor, Department of Surgery, University of California, San Francisco, San Francisco, California, USA

DAVID T. FETZER, MD
Department of Radiology, University of Texas Southwestern Medical Center, Dallas, Texas, USA

CESAR GARCIA, BS
Department of Neurosurgery, Stanford School of Medicine, Stanford, California, USA

MICHAEL H. GERBER, MD
CT Fellow, Department of Surgery, Section of Thoracic Surgery, University of Arizona, Tucson, Arizona, USA

KENT GOODMAN
Division of Surgical Oncology, Department of Surgery, University of California, San Francisco, San Francisco, California, USA

CLAIRE E. GRAVES, MD
Assistant Professor, Section of Endocrine Surgery, Department of Surgery, University of California, Davis, Sacramento, California, USA

H. HENRY GUO, MD, PhD
Clinical Associate Professor, Department of Radiology, Stanford University, Stanford, California, USA

MELANIE HAYDEN-GEPHART, MAS, MD
Masters of Advanced Sciences, Department of Neurosurgery, Stanford School of Medicine, Stanford, California, USA

MARISA HOM, PhD
Department of Otolaryngology–Head and Neck Surgery, Vanderbilt University Medical Center, Nashville, Tennessee, USA

SHRUTI JAIN, PhD
Department of Neurosurgery, Stanford School of Medicine, Stanford, California, USA

ELLA F. JONES, PhD
Department of Radiology and Biomedical Imaging, University of California, San Francisco, San Francisco, California, USA

LILY KIM, MD
Department of Neurosurgery, Stanford School of Medicine, Stanford, California, USA

KATE KRAUSE, MD
Fellow in Cardiothoracic Surgery, Division of Thoracic Surgery, Massachusetts General Hospital, Boston, Massachusetts, USA

JENNIFER J. KWAK, MD
Associate Professor, Department of Radiology, School of Medicine, University of Colorado, Aurora, Colorado, USA

COURTNEY LAWHN-HEATH, MD
Department of Radiology and Biomedical Imaging, University of California, San Francisco, San Francisco, California, USA

GUAN LI, BS
Department of Neurosurgery, Stanford School of Medicine, Stanford, California, USA

NATALIE S. LUI, MD, MAS
Assistant Professor of Cardiothoracic Surgery, Stanford School of Medicine, Stanford, California, USA

NADINE MALLAK, MD
Associate Professor of Diagnostic Radiology, Oregon Health & Science University, Portland, Oregon, USA

LUCAS MANI, MS
Department of Otolaryngology–Head and Neck Surgery, Vanderbilt University Medical Center, Nashville, Tennessee, USA

ESTELLE MARTIN
Department of Otolaryngology–Head and Neck Surgery, Vanderbilt University Medical Center, Nashville, Tennessee, USA

JULISSA MOLINA-VEGA, BA
Division of Surgical Oncology, Department of Surgery, University of California, San Francisco, San Francisco, California, USA

RITA A. MUKHTAR, MD
Division of Surgical Oncology, Department of Surgery, University of California, San Francisco, San Francisco, California, USA

EUNKYUNG ANGELA PARK, MD, PhD
Clinical Assistant Professor, Division of Nuclear Medicine, Department of Radiology, University of Iowa Hospitals and Clinics, Iowa City, Iowa, USA

MATTHEW R. POREMBKA, MD
Associate Professor, Division of Surgical Oncology, Dedman Family Scholar in Clinical Care, The University of Texas Southwestern Medical Center, Dallas, Texas, USA

ADRIAN RODRIGUES, BA
Department of Neurosurgery, Stanford School of Medicine, Stanford, California, USA

EBEN L. ROSENTHAL, MD
Department of Otolaryngology–Head and Neck Surgery, Vanderbilt University Medical Center, Nashville, Tennessee, USA

UMA M. SACHDEVA, MD, PhD
Assistant Professor of Surgery, Division of Thoracic Surgery, Massachusetts General Hospital and Harvard Medical School, Boston, Massachusetts, USA

LANA Y. SCHUMACHER, MD
Assistant Professor of Surgery, Division of Thoracic Surgery, Massachusetts General Hospital and Harvard Medical School, Boston, Massachusetts, USA

SUNIL SINGHAL, MD
Chief, Division of Thoracic Surgery, Vice Chair, Translational Research, Department of Surgery, William Maul Measey Professor in Surgical Research, University of Pennsylvania, Philadelphia, Pennsylvania, USA

INSOO SUH, MD
Associate Professor and Associate Vice Chair of Surgical Innovation, Department of Surgery, NYU Langone Health, New York, New York, USA

LASZLO SZIDONYA, MD, PhD
Diagnostic Radiology Fellow, Oregon Health & Science University, Portland, Oregon, USA; Assistant Professor, Diagnostic Radiology, Heart and Vascular Center, Semmelweis University, Budapest, Hungary

STEPHANIE G. WORRELL, MD, FACS
Assistant Professor, Department of Surgery, Section of Thoracic Surgery, University of Arizona, Tucson, Arizona, USA

MICHAEL ZHANG, MD
Department of Neurosurgery, Stanford School of Medicine, Stanford, California, USA

Contents

 Video content accompanies this article at http://www.surgonc. theclinics.com.

[18]F-fluoroestradiol (^{18}F-FES) is a Food and Drug Administration-approved radiopharmaceutical used for molecular imaging of the estrogen receptor (ER). When combined with PET, ^{18}F-FES may improve the diagnosis of ER-positive breast cancer in the metastatic setting and provide insights into tumor heterogeneity. In this article, we review data on the use of ^{18}F-FES imaging for treatment selection, staging, imaging lobular breast cancer, and the novel breast specific imaging tool, dedicated breast PET.

 Video content accompanies this article at http://www.surgonc. theclinics.com.

High-grade glioma is the most common malignant primary brain tumor in adults. Glioma infiltration renders it difficult to treat and likely to recur. Increasing the extent of resection has been associated with improving progression-free survival and overall survival by several months. The introduction of 5-aminolevulinic acid (5-ALA) fluorescence-guided surgery has allowed surgeons to better differentiate between neoplastic tissue and normal tissue, thus achieving greater extent of resection. The development of new intraoperative imaging modalities in combination with 5-ALA may provide additional benefits for glioma patients.

Pulmonary segmentectomy has become a widely accepted technique for resection of early-stage lung cancers. Intraoperative identification of small nodules within the lung parenchyma and definition of segmental anatomy are essential for oncologic segmental resection and significantly enhanced by recent advances in imaging techniques. Advances in imaging for nodule localization, using preoperative markers and three-dimensional computed tomography, delineation of segmental anatomy, and sentinel lymph node mapping have become important components of planning and performing minimally invasive anatomic segmentectomies and are particularly well suited for the evolving robotic-assisted platform.

During an esophagectomy, many factors influence the anastomosis. Surgical factors include anastomotic tension, location of the anastomosis, surgical technique, and perfusion of the conduit. The use of fluorescent angiography is a possible avenue for more objective evaluation of the gastric conduit. There is a lot of variability in the way this tool has been used and what the results indicate. This article will discuss the various methods of fluorescent angiography to determine intestinal perfusion using indocyanine green and fluorescent imaging and the data on the association with clinical outcomes.

During cervical surgery, localization and identification of parathyroid glands is key to both the removal of abnormal hyperfunctioning glands and the preservation of normal glands. The challenging nature of parathyroid localization has fostered innovation in imaging techniques to localize glands both before and during cervical operations. Advances in preoperative imaging include PET-based imaging modalities paired with computed tomography or MRI for anatomic correlation. During surgery, both parathyroid autofluorescence and contrast-enhanced fluorescence techniques are useful adjuncts for intraoperative identification.

Positron emission tomography (PET) with somatostatin receptor (SSTR) ligands has taken the lead in the imaging of neuroendocrine tumors (NETs). In this article, we review the role of SSTR PET scan in the management of NETs, including the indications for the scan, pitfalls in interpretation, and imaging selection criteria for peptide receptor radionuclide therapy. We also discuss the complementary role of fluorodeoxyglucose PET particularly for patients with high-grade disease.

A variety of three-dimensional (3D) printing techniques and materials facilitate the creation of customized models that promise to improve surgical procedures and patient outcomes. Three-dimensional-printed models allow patients, trainees, and experienced surgeons to explore anatomy through direct visualization and tactile feedback. Although 3D-printed models serve a range of purposes including preoperative planning, education, skills refinement, patient-specific intraprocedural guides, and implants, much work remains to decrease the turnaround time and cost of printing models, collect long-term effectiveness data, and refine regulatory oversight of 3D printing in medicine.

Intraoperative molecular imaging shows great promise in the surgical treatment of lung cancer, in particular tumor localization, margin assessment, identification of additional nodules, and even potentially lymph node assessment. Advances in imaging agents and fluorescence surgical cameras will be the key. Although no imaging agent is currently Food and Drug Administration approved, targeted, near-infrared agents such as OTL38 are in phase III trials.

Despite improvements in medical management of head and neck cancers, positive surgical margin rates have remained relatively unchanged in the past 30 years, emphasizing a need for improved intraoperative imaging and tumor visualization. This review provides a detailed summary on preoperative anatomic imaging techniques, nonspecific fluorescence imaging modalities, the recent emergence of tumor-targeting fluorophores for intraoperative imaging, and the future of fluorescence-guided surgery in head and neck cancer.

Contrast-enhanced intraoperative ultrasound (CE-IOUS) is a relatively new but valuable tool that is increasingly used as an adjunct to computed tomography, MRI, and IOUS for patients undergoing liver surgery. CE-IOUS has an important role in 2 main settings: the discrimination of indeterminate lesions detected in cirrhotic livers by conventional IOUS and in the detection of colorectal liver metastasis that may be overlooked by other imaging modalities. The intraoperative nature of the imaging and interpretation allows for CE-IOUS to directly affect surgical decision-making that may importantly affect patient outcomes.

SURGICAL ONCOLOGY CLINICS OF NORTH AMERICA

SERIES OF RELATED INTEREST

Advances in Surgery
https://www.advancessurgery.com
Surgical Clinics of North America
https://www.surgical.theclinics.com
Thoracic Surgery Clinics
https://www.thoracic.theclinics.com

THE CLINICS ARE AVAILABLE ONLINE!
Access your subscription at:
www.theclinics.com

Foreword

Oncology Imaging: Updates and Advancements

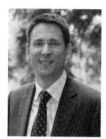

Timothy M. Pawlik, MD, PhD, MPH, MTS, MBA, FACS, FSSO, RACS (Hon.)
Consulting Editor

This issue of the *Surgical Oncology Clinics of North America* focuses on updates and advancements in oncology imaging.

Imaging plays a pivotal role in the multidisciplinary treatment of virtually every single patient with patient. In fact, the use of imaging can be argued to form the basis of almost every clinical decision: screening, diagnosis, operative/treatment planning, assessment of response, as well as ongoing surveillance. Recent advances in imaging have involved improved technology and techniques related to cross-sectional imaging, as well as novel applications of functional imaging and the merging of therapeutics with targeted imaging agents. Future advances in imaging hold the promise of further integration of morphologic, structural, metabolic, and functional information to assist in clinical decision making, as well as application of novel radiomic data to inform cancer care. As imaging modalities and technology have evolved, so have our need to understand better how to integrate these news tools into clinical practice. In particular, the surgeon plays a central role in the use and application of imaging as related to the patient with cancer. As such, I am grateful to have Natalie S. Lui, MD, MAS as the guest editor of this important issue of *Surgical Oncology Clinics of North America*. Dr Lui is assistant professor at Stanford University School of Medicine. Dr Lui studied physics as an undergraduate at Harvard before attending medical school at Johns Hopkins. She completed a general surgery residency at the University of California San Francisco (UCSF), which included 2 years of research in the UCSF Thoracic Oncology Laboratory and completion of a Master's in Advanced Studies in clinical research. Dr Lui went on to hold a fellowship in Thoracic Surgery at Massachusetts General Hospital, during which time she participated in visiting rotations at Memorial Sloan Kettering and the Mayo Clinic. Dr Lui's surgical practice consists of general thoracic surgery with a focus on thoracic oncology and robotic thoracic surgery. Her research interests include intraoperative molecular imaging for lung cancer

Surg Oncol Clin N Am 31 (2022) xi–xii
https://doi.org/10.1016/j.soc.2022.07.011
1055-3207/22/© 2022 Published by Elsevier Inc.

localization, increasing rates of lung cancer screening, and using artificial intelligence to predict lung cancer recurrence. As such, Dr Lui is imminently qualified to be the guest editor of this important issue of *Surgical Oncology Clinics of North America*.

The issue covers a number of important topics that focus on state-of-the-art imaging updates across a wide range of oncologic diseases. In particular, an extraordinary team of experts detail various imaging updates related to tumors, including breast cancer, malignant glioma, parathyroid disease, and, among others, neuroendocrine tumors. In addition, other important topics that are relevant to surgeons, such as intraoperative molecular imaging, intraoperative ultrasound, as well as 3D reconstruction and printing to aid in surgical planning, are covered.

I wish to express my sincere gratitude to Dr Lui for her work to identify such a wonderful group of oncology leaders with expertise in cancer-related imaging to contribute to this issue of *Surgical Oncology Clinics of North America*. This team of authors has done a masterful job emphasizing the important and relevant aspects of imaging in cancer care. I know that this issue of *Surgical Oncology Clinics of North America* will serve trainees and faculty well in acquainting them with the latest up-to-date data on oncology imaging. I would like to thank Dr Lui and all the expert authors again for an outstanding issue of the *Surgical Oncology Clinics of North America*.

Timothy M. Pawlik, MD, PhD, MPH, MTS, MBA, FACS, FSSO, RACS (Hon.)
Department of Surgery
The Ohio State University
Wexner Medical Center
395 West 12th Avenue, Suite 670
Columbus, OH 43210, USA

E-mail address:
tim.pawlik@osumc.edu

Preface

Oncology Imaging: Updates and Advancements

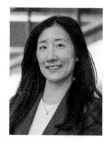

Natalie S. Lui, MD, MAS
Editor

Imaging is at the core of surgical oncology. Longstanding techniques, such as computed tomography and MRI, as well as nuclear medicine methods, such as PET, have been studied and refined over the years. They form the basis of preoperative staging and complex surgical planning. For a long time, surgeons relied on these preoperative scans, and there was little imaging performed intraoperatively to guide surgical resection.

Recently, there has been an explosion in new imaging techniques and methods. Many of these, such as microbubble contrast for liver ultrasound, are used intraoperatively to guide surgical resection. Several new fluorescence imaging agents are used intraoperatively for tumor localization and margin assessment. Some of these, such as indocyanine green, are nontargeted and work in a variety of tumors. Others, such as 5-aminolevulinic acid, are used in the specific tumors in which they accumulate. Additional imaging agents, such as fluoroestradiol, are used perioperatively to improve tumor identification and plan systemic therapy.

This issue contains a sample of the exciting innovations in surgical oncology imaging, some established clinically, some recently introduced, and some in the pipeline and close to approval. The articles cover a wide range of imaging techniques in a variety of malignancies. They demonstrate the vitality of this field that is welcomed by surgeons looking to improve their operative techniques and oncologic outcomes. The articles also cover some of the limitations to these new approaches, including additional time and cost, as well as surgeon training.

I hope you enjoy reading about the latest updates and advancements in imaging across a wide range of surgical oncology subspecialties. And I look forward to seeing

Surg Oncol Clin N Am 31 (2022) xiii–xiv
https://doi.org/10.1016/j.soc.2022.07.012
1055-3207/22/© 2022 Published by Elsevier Inc.

these techniques developed further to help the surgical management of our patients in the future.

Natalie S. Lui, MD, MAS
Stanford University School of Medicine
300 Pasteur Drive
Falk Building
Stanford, CA 94305, USA

E-mail address:
natalielui@stanford.edu

Molecular Imaging for Estrogen Receptor-Positive Breast Cancer

Clinical Applications of Whole Body and Dedicated Breast Positron Emission Tomography

Kent Goodman[a,1], Mary Kathryn Abel, AB[b,1], Courtney Lawhn-Heath, MD[c], Julissa Molina-Vega, BA[a], Ella F. Jones, PhD[c], Rita A. Mukhtar, MD[a,*]

KEYWORDS

- Fluoroestradiol • Molecular imaging • Breast cancer • Lobular breast cancer
- Staging • Positron emission tomography

KEY POINTS

- ^{18}F-Fluoroestradiol (^{18}F-FES) is a radiopharmaceutical for molecular imaging of ER + breast cancers
- Baseline ^{18}F-FES uptake may be used to guide treatment strategies
- Molecular imaging may improve disease staging

Continued

 Video content accompanies this article at http://www.surgonc.theclinics.com.

INTRODUCTION

An estimated 3.5 million women in the United States are living with breast cancer, with nearly 290,000 new cases expected in 2022.[1] During the past several decades, there

Funding: R.A. Mukhtar was supported by the National Cancer Institute Award K08CA256047. E. F. Jones was supported in part by the Department of Defense W81XWH-18-1-0671 and National Institutes of Health R01CA227763.
[a] Division of Surgical Oncology, Department of Surgery, University of California, San Francisco, 1825 4th Street, 3rd Floor, Box 1710, San Francisco, CA 94143, USA; [b] School of Medicine, University of California, San Francisco, 505 Parnassus Avenue San Francisco, CA 94143, USA; [c] Department of Radiology and Biomedical Imaging, University of California, San Francisco, 505 Parnassus Avenue San Francisco, CA 94143, USA
[1] Contributed equally to this article.
* Corresponding author.
E-mail address: rita.mukhtar@ucsf.edu

Surg Oncol Clin N Am 31 (2022) 569–579
https://doi.org/10.1016/j.soc.2022.06.001
1055-3207/22/© 2022 Elsevier Inc. All rights reserved.

Continued

- Dedicated breast positron emission tomography scanning with ^{18}F-FES may provide more accurate tumor assessments in early-stage disease, and noninvasive therapy response indicators
- Estrogen receptor (ER) modulators and degraders will block ^{18}F-FES binding, and should be held for a minimum of 6 to 8 weeks selective ER modulators or 28 weeks selective ER downregulators/degraders before imaging to avoid false negatives

have been significant strides in breast cancer diagnosis and management. The appreciation for tumor subtypes defined by receptor status has fundamentally changed our understanding of breast cancer and is used to direct treatment strategies. For estrogen receptor-positive (ER+) tumors, treatment with endocrine therapy such as ER modulators or aromatase inhibitors dramatically improves outcomes.[2] For those with overexpression or amplification of the human epidermal growth factor receptor-2 (HER-2), targeted treatment with HER-2 antibody-based therapy is now standard.[3]

For many years, investigators have studied whether these receptors can also be used for imaging breast tumors.[4,5] Such targeted molecular imaging has the promise of improved tumor detection, potentially determination of response to therapy, and could guide treatment strategies and improve surgical approaches. The imaging agent ^{18}F-fluoroestradiol (^{18}F-FES) is a PET radiopharmaceutical used for noninvasive imaging of the ER in vivo. In this article, we discuss the history and development of ^{18}F-FES PET, its clinical applications, its potential utility in invasive lobular carcinoma (ILC), and its use with the novel imaging tool, dedicated breast PET (dbPET).

DISCUSSION
History and Development of ^{18}F-Fluoroestradiol

The development of ^{18}F-FES is largely credited to Dr John A. Katzenellenbogen, a chemist from the University of Illinois. His early study began by efforts to obtain gamma-emitting estrogens, specifically using radioiodinated steroidal estrogens with estradiol substituted at the 16α-position. Guided by the study of Dr Richard Hochberg, who found that 16α-[^{125}I]iodoestradiol had better ER-binding affinities in vivo, Katzenellenbogen began experimenting with other radioisotopes substituted at the 16α-position. Eventually, his team identified that 16α-[[77]Br]bromoestradiol had improved binding over 16α-[^{125}I]iodoestradiol, but translation from rats to humans proved disappointing.[6] A change in isotope to fluorine-18 allowed the team to benefit from the timely progress in PET imaging technology. The team prepared a variety of [^{18}F]-labeled steroidal and nonsteroidal estrogens but focusing on the 16α-[^{18}F]-FES in particular, which they named ^{18}F-FES. In 1984, Katzenellenbogen and his team first reported favorable biodistribution characteristics of ^{18}F-FES in rats, and the first images of ER + breast tumors in human subjects were published in 1988.[7] Subsequent years have seen studies evaluating the technical validity, clinical validity, and clinical utility of ^{18}F-FES in the diagnosis and management of breast cancer, with more studies ongoing.[8] Approval from the US Food and Drug Administration (FDA) for its use in recurrent or metastatic ER + breast cancers in conjunction with biopsy was received in May 2020.

Clinical Applications of ^{18}F-Fluoroestradiol in Breast Cancer

^{18}F-FES has binding affinity for the ER, ranging from 60% to 100% across reported studies.[9–11] As such, when paired with standard imaging procedures such as PET

and computed tomography (CT), ^{18}F-FES can serve as a "noninvasive whole-body biopsy" to identify ER+ lesions.[9]

^{18}F-FES is administered intravenously over 1 to 2 minutes, with PET image acquisition occurring after a 30 to 100-minute uptake period, with imaging at 80 minutes recommended.[9,12–15] The agent is metabolized by the liver and excreted through the biliary tract into the small bowel, with additional excretion by the kidneys. Of note, physiologic uptake is more pronounced in liver and small bowel than kidney and bladder.[16] Ligand quantities are low enough to avoid physiological effects.[17] Because ^{18}F-FES binds to the ER, the use of ER antagonists or degraders results in decreased ^{18}F-FES PET signal.[18] The currently recommended washout period before imaging with ^{18}F-FES is 8 weeks for selective ER modulators (SERMs) and 28 weeks for selective ER downregulators/degraders (SERDs). As a result, repeat ^{18}F-FES PET imaging is generally only feasible in patients not on SERMs or SERDs.

Detection of estrogen receptor

There have been several studies suggesting a strong correlation between ^{18}F-FES uptake and ER positivity as measured by immunohistochemistry (IHC). Compared with IHC, ^{18}F-FES PET was found to have a pooled sensitivity of 82% and specificity of 95% for ER positivity in a meta-analysis of 9 prospective studies.[19] A more recent meta-analysis evaluating the ability of FES to determine ER status of breast and non-breast lesions in patients with metastatic breast cancer found an overall sensitivity of 81% and specificity of 85%.[20] **Fig. 1** demonstrates a left breast cancer visible on dynamic contrast-enhanced MRI, with no uptake on ^{18}F-FES PET, consistent with biopsy-proven ER-negative status. One study found that ^{18}F-FES had a positive predictive value of 100% and a negative predictive value of 78%, which changed depending on the threshold of the maximum standardized uptake value (SUV_{max}),[12] with the caveat that patients with bone metastases were excluded. In this study, the authors suggest that tumors that are ER + on IHC but negative on ^{18}F-FES PET might reflect the lack of ER functionality as opposed to a false-negative imaging test; more investigation into this hypothesis is needed.

Although IHC analysis remains the gold standard for determining the presence of ER, there are benefits of ^{18}F-FES over biopsy alone. One potential advantage to ^{18}F-FES is the ability to noninvasively assay the whole tumor, providing a more comprehensive assessment of functional ER status than IHC of a limited tumor sample. Evaluation of

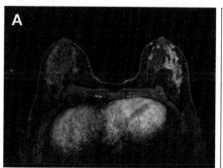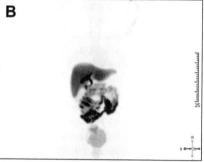

Fig. 1. Patient with left breast multicentric left breast ER-negative, progesterone receptor-negative, HER 2-positive IDC. (*A*) shows dynamic contrast-enhanced MRI showing extensive mass and nonmass enhancement in outer left breast. In (*B*), ^{18}F-FES PET scan shows no uptake in left breast, consistent with ER negativity of known tumor, with expected uptake in liver and gastrointestinal tract.

^{18}F-FES uptake within a tumor could reflect intratumoral heterogeneity not elucidated from biopsy alone. Moreover, receptor status may not be uniform across all tumors in a given patient with metastatic disease. Yang and colleagues showed that 37.5% of patients with metastatic breast cancer presented with both ER+ and ER-disease, which may or may not be identified based on biopsy alone, depending on the number of sites biopsied. ^{18}F-FES, however, can help identify metastatic lesions based on the uptake of the tracer in a single test, which has the potential to guide treatment, improve response to therapy, and perhaps even prolong survival.[9] Additionally, whole-body ^{18}F-FES PET can be used to evaluate multiple lesions in a noninvasive manner, including sites such as the brain that would be challenging to biopsy. In fact, imaging of brain metastases is of particular clinical interest because PET scanning using fluorodeoxyglucose (FDG-PET) can be limited due to the high FDG avidity of normal cerebral cortex and deep gray nuclei.[21] In one study by Ivanidze and colleagues[21], ^{18}F-FES brain PET/CT demonstrated increased avidity in a brain lesion suggesting metastatic disease, although also showing decreased avidity in a lesion that was thought to represent posttreatment change.

Systemic therapy selection

One of the proposed clinical applications for ^{18}F-FES is for therapy selection. Some of the initial studies assessing ^{18}F-FES and treatment response were in patients with advanced breast cancer treated with tamoxifen.[22–24] Mortimer and colleagues[23] postulated that ^{18}F-FES PET could be used to identify hormonally responsive cancers. In their pivotal 2011 study, the authors found that the functional status of ER can be determined using ^{18}F-FES PET and can predict response to tamoxifen. In another study of 51 patients with advanced ER + breast cancer, higher baseline ^{18}F-FES uptake was predictive of response to tamoxifen; additionally, a detectable "metabolic flare" on FDG-PET after estradiol challenge was observed in patients who were more responsive to tamoxifen.[25] Indeed, combining characteristics of tumors on both ^{18}F-FES and FDG-PET may allow for further patient stratification.[26]

In the metastatic setting, disease with low uptake of ^{18}F-FES has been associated with worse response to endocrine treatment, with a cohort study of 47 patients with pretreated metastatic breast cancer identifying a threshold SUV of less than 1.5 being predictive of lack of response.[24] Interestingly, van Kruchten and colleagues[27] found that although baseline ^{18}F-FES uptake was not associated with disease progression, the persistence of uptake on follow-up ^{18}F-FES PET after SERD initiation was associated with earlier progression, possibly indicating incomplete ER degradation.

^{18}F-FES has also been used to assess potential benefit of other therapeutic agents used in metastatic breast cancer, including cyclin-dependent kinase (CDK) inhibitors. Although adding CDK inhibitors to endocrine treatment has been shown to improve invasive disease-free survival in some patients with metastatic ER + breast cancer, better understanding of ER heterogeneity could potentially improve patient selection for treatment.[28] In a prospective analysis of 30 patients with metastatic ER + breast cancer, ER heterogeneity was determined by measuring what proportion of lesions visible on either FDG-PET or CT were avid on ^{18}F-FES PET.[29] Those with the highest proportion of ^{18}F-FES-positive disease at baseline had the longest time to progression on combination endocrine therapy with CDK4/6 inhibition. Additionally, those with better response to combination treatment, as measured by reduced lesion metabolic activity on FDG-PET, had higher ^{18}F-FES uptake. These findings suggest that combining ^{18}F-FES imaging with other imaging modalities can be used to differentiate among those with ER-positive disease and identify heterogeneous disease patterns that might benefit from differing treatment strategies.

A novel potential application of ¹⁸F-FES imaging includes determining whether resistance to endocrine therapy has been overcome. In a recent study, histone deacetylase inhibition with vorinostat was used with the goal of restoring endocrine therapy sensitivity in 23 patients with metastatic ER + breast cancer.[30] Although subsequent ¹⁸F-FES PET imaging did not show increased uptake compared with baseline to indicate restored ER ligand binding, higher baseline ¹⁸F-FES uptake was again associated with improved progression free survival.[30] The authors note, however, that although ¹⁸F-FES uptake indicates the ability of the ER to bind ligand, this is not necessarily indicative of endocrine therapy sensitivity, particularly given multiple pathways influencing such sensitivity, and challenges with the definition of sensitivity which may differ by disease site (eg, disease progression in visceral versus bone metastases). However, achieving complete blockade or suppression of ER as measured by lack of ¹⁸F-FES uptake on known ER + lesions has been reported for purposes of finding optimal doses for ER-modulating agents.[31]

Resolving clinical dilemmas

¹⁸F-FES PET may be useful in patients with ER + breast cancer who present with clinical dilemmas where conventional workup is inconclusive. For example, a Dutch study included patients with metastatic breast cancer whose staging imaging, including CT chest/abdomen/pelvis, abdominal ultrasound, and bone scan, yielded equivocal findings.[32] ¹⁸F-FES PET was most sensitive for bone metastases and improved diagnostic understanding in 88% of patients, leading to a change in therapy in 48% of those patients. Similar results were presented by Sun and colleagues,[33] who found that ¹⁸F-FES PET aided the diagnosis and changed treatment plans in approximately half of patients in their study. **Fig. 2** demonstrates imaging findings from a patient with

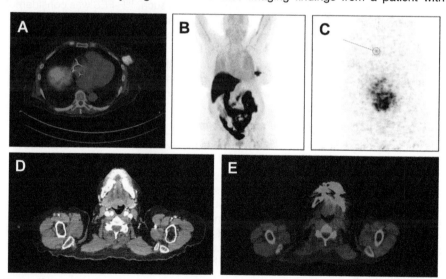

Fig. 2. ¹⁸F-FES imaging in patient with left breast ER-positive HER2-negative ILC and oropharyngeal mass for which nondiagnostic biopsy had been performed. (*A*) Shows left breast mass with ¹⁸F-FES uptake on fused PET-CT reflecting ER positivity. (*B*) Shows 18-F PET highlighting tumor in left breast, with expected uptake of ¹⁸F-FES in liver and gastrointestinal tract. In (*C*), left breast is imaged with dedicated breast PET using 18-F FES, identifying a possible satellite lesion anterior to known tumor. Finally, (*D*) shows image from CT scan demonstrating irregular oropharyngeal mass, and fused image from 18-F FES PET-CT (*E*) shows no uptake in mass, suggesting that this mass was unrelated to primary ILC tumor.

biopsy-proven ER + ILC of the left breast with imaging studies identifying an oropha-ryngeal lesion of unclear cause despite attempted biopsy; this case illustrates the potential additive role of ^{18}F-FES PET for clinical decision-making.

The Use of ^{18}F-Fluoroestradiol in Invasive Lobular Carcinoma of the Breast

Although ^{18}F-FES PET may have wide applicability in the diagnosis and management of breast cancer, there are certain subtypes of breast cancer that may benefit even more from this technology. One such subtype is ILC. ILC is the second most common type of breast cancer, accounting for 10% to 15% of all patients with breast cancer. Due to the infiltrative growth pattern of ILC compared with the more common invasive ductal carcinoma (IDC), it is often harder to detect with standard imaging modalities, including FDG-PET. Moreover, nearly 95% of all lobular cancers are ER positive. As such, ^{18}F-FES PET is promising for the evaluation of this breast cancer subtype.

One of the first studies to evaluate the use of ^{18}F-FES PET in ILC was a case series by Venema and colleagues in 2017.[34] The authors reported 3 lobular breast cancer cases, where confirmation of metastatic disease was imperative for subsequent treatment, and biopsy was not possible. In these 3 cases, standard imaging modalities such as CT, MRI, and FDG-PET returned equivocal results, whereas ^{18}F-FES PET provided definitive diagnosis of metastatic lesions. The authors concluded that ^{18}F-FES PET may have added value compared with conventional staging mechanisms.

Further studies have compared the use of ^{18}F-FES versus FDG-PET in the diagnosis of metastatic ILC. Ulaner and colleagues[35] evaluated results from 7 patients with ILC who underwent both ^{18}F-FES and FDG-PET imaging. The authors found that ^{18}F-FES detected more metastatic lesions in patients with ILC compared to FDG-PET, and no patients presented with only FDG-avid metastases. As such, ^{18}F-FES was considered to compare favorably to FDG for assessing metastases in ILC patients. **Fig. 3** illustrates a case of de novo metastatic ER + ILC in which additional lesions were seen on ^{18}F-FES PET compared with FDG-PET.

Given the predilection of ILC for a diffuse growth pattern, further research is needed to assess the use of ^{18}F-FES PET in settings of poorly visualized disease, including peritoneal carcinomatosis, leptomeningeal disease, and pleural effusions.

Challenges in the Implementation of ^{18}F-FES Imaging Studies

One of the primary limitations of ^{18}F-FES PET is the evaluation of liver metastases. As described previously, there is a high level of normal physiologic uptake of ^{18}F-FES in the liver resulting from rapid metabolism of the agent. This issue led one research group to conclude that ^{18}F-FES PET should not be used to evaluate liver metastases.[34] However, a recent article by Boers and colleagues sought to evaluate whether ^{18}F-FES could be used to identify ER + liver metastases, confirmed by biopsy, comparing visual and quantitative measures, and evaluating the impact of modifying region of interest. Although quantitative analysis improved sensitivity of detection over visual analysis, specificity was reduced.[36] Currently, ^{18}F-FES PET may have limited clinical utility in the detection of liver metastases.

An additional concern about ^{18}F-FES PET is the cost when compared with biopsy alone, assuming that biopsy is feasible. There has been only one cost-effectiveness model that has been published to date about the use of ^{18}F-FES in metastatic breast cancer, which was based on hospitals within the Dutch health-care system.[37] Although more metastatic lesions were identified using ^{18}F-FES PET, the diagnostic costs to evaluate receptor status and treatment costs were higher compared with biopsy alone.

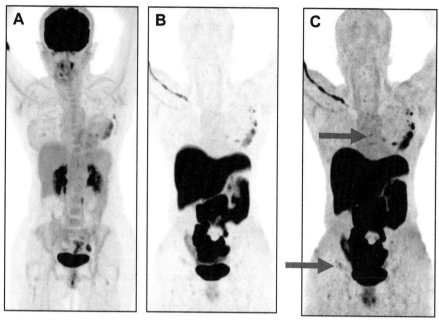

Fig. 3. Patient with left breast palpable ER-positive HER2-negative ILC with de novo stage IV disease. Panel A shows FDG-PET with uptake at known left breast mass. (*B, C*) show 18-F FES PET demonstrating foci of low-level avidity on rewindowing images for higher sensitivity, consistent with bone metastases. Bone metastases in sternum and iliac crest denoted by red *arrows*.

As with many PET radiotracers, ^{18}F-FES uptake quantitation can be influenced by body mass index, with higher body mass index being associated with increased uptake; this can be overcome by correcting quantitative measurements for lean body mass.[38] Additionally, many ER + lesions have a low tumor to background ratio; the low SUV$_{max}$ threshold for positivity on ^{18}F-FES PET can pose a sensitivity challenge in FES PET image interpretation.

Dedicated Breast Positron Emission Tomography and ^{18}F-Fluoroestradiol

Although the literature contains many studies evaluating the use of ^{18}F-FES with whole-body PET imaging, dbPET is a promising new technology that may be a complementary tool. Imaging the breast only, dbPET provides higher resolution of breast lesions than whole-body PET, and it may be especially relevant for the evaluation of early stage disease and surgical planning.

Compared with whole-body PET, dbPET uses a lower dose of radiotracer (185 vs 370 MBq) and less radiation, potentially allowing more opportunities for serial imaging.[39] Moreover, the positioning of the patient prone rather than supine in dbPET prevents breast compression, thereby allowing full breast volume imaging akin to breast MRI. dbPET has demonstrated higher sensitivity in detecting subcentimeter lesions and may identify response to neoadjuvant chemotherapy earlier than MRI.[40] Importantly, however, this high sensitivity comes with the possibility of detecting benign lesions and higher false-positive rates.[41] Recently, there has been a push to standardize reporting and descriptors of uptake in dbPET given its increasing use.[41]

The literature evaluating the use of ^{18}F-FES in dbPET is extremely limited. One feasibility study by Jones and colleagues[40] outlined their initial experiences with dbPET using

^{18}F-FES in assessing ER + breast cancer in 6 patients, including 2 with ILC. The results suggest the potential of ^{18}F-FES PET imaging to provide early predictions of neoadjuvant treatment efficacy and thus aid in therapy selection. The authors also noted important limitations to the technology, including variations in ^{18}F-FES uptake in different ER-positive breast cancer subtypes and the exclusion of axillary lymph nodes.[40]

Future Directions

As of this writing, ^{18}F-FES PET is FDA-approved for imaging ER-positive lesions as an adjunct to biopsy in patients with recurrent or metastatic breast cancer. However, ^{18}F-FES PET could be used as a beneficial adjunct to FDG-PET and other diagnostic imaging modalities to aid in initial staging.[42] In particular, ^{18}F-FES may be able to reduce false-positive FDG-PET results caused by inflammation or improve staging in difficult to detect tumors such as ILC, as described above.[42,43]

Currently, there is an open clinical trial evaluating the use of ^{18}F-FES for staging and detection of recurrent ER-positive breast cancer compared with standard of care with chest, abdominal, and pelvic CT and bone scan (NCT04883814).[44] Other ongoing trials evaluating the clinical utility of ^{18}F-FES include the ECOG-ACRIN EAI 142 trial (NCT02398773), a phase II study of patients with ER + metastatic breast cancer prospectively evaluating ^{18}F-FES PET as a predictor of clinical benefit and progression free survival to first-line endocrine therapy. Similarly, the ongoing ET-FES TRANSCAN trial (EUDRACT 2013–000–287–29) is testing tumoral heterogeneity on ^{18}F-FES PET as a predictor of endocrine therapy response.[45] The Imaging Patients for Cancer Drug Selection – Metastatic Breast Cancer study (NCT01957332) tests the clinical utility of ^{18}F-FES PET for reducing biopsies and improving treatment selection. Results from these results may solidify ^{18}F-FES's place in staging and detection of recurrent breast cancer, and treatment selection for metastatic disease.

With increased resolution compared with whole body PET, dbPET may prove useful in accurate assessment of breast tumor size, facilitating surgical planning, and potentially reducing the need for re-excisions. In addition, dbPET may be a useful adjunct to MRI for assessing response to neoadjuvant therapy.

SUMMARY

Recently FDA-approved, ^{18}F-FES is a well-studied radiopharmaceutical with the ability to provide molecular imaging of ER-positive breast cancer. In the setting of whole-body PET scanning, ^{18}F-FES uptake can confirm the presence of ER + metastases and provide insight into tumor heterogeneity. Uptake values may reflect sensitivity to therapy and guide treatment selection. In the setting of ILC, ^{18}F-FES may provide improved disease detection compared with standard FDG-PET. The novel dedicated breast PET technology may provide improved tumor resolution that can be used both for evaluating the response to neoadjuvant treatment and for providing more accurate staging for surgical planning.

DISCLOSURE

No disclosures for all authors included in this article.

REFERENCES

1. Breast cancer facts and statistics. Available at: https://www.breastcancer.org/facts-statistics. Accessed March 6, 2022.

2. Carlson RW, Hudis CA, Pritchard KI. National comprehensive cancer network breast cancer clinical practice guidelines in oncology, american society of clinical oncology technology assessment on the use of aromatase inhibitors, St Gallen international expert consensus on the primary therapy of early breast cancer. Adjuvant endocrine therapy in hormone receptor-positive postmenopausal breast cancer: evolution of NCCN, ASCO, and St Gallen recommendations. J Natl Compr Cancer Netw 2006;4(10):971–9.

3. Brown-Glaberman U, Dayao Z, Royce M. HER2-targeted therapy for early-stage breast cancer: a comprehensive review. Oncol Williston Park N 2014;28(4): 281–9.

4. Li H, Liu Z, Yuan L, et al. Radionuclide-based imaging of breast cancer: state of the art. Cancers 2021;13(21):5459.

5. Linden HM, Dehdashti F. Novel methods and tracers for breast cancer imaging. Semin Nucl Med 2013;43(4):324–9.

6. McElvany KD, Katzenellenbogen JA, Shafer KE, et al. 16 alpha-[77Br] bromoestradiol: dosimetry and preliminary clinical studies. J Nucl Med 1982; 23(5):425–30.

7. Mintun MA, Welch MJ, Siegel BA, et al. Breast cancer: PET imaging of estrogen receptors. Radiology 1988;169(1):45–8.

8. Boers J, de Vries EFJ, Glaudemans AWJM, et al. Application of PET tracers in molecular imaging for breast cancer. Curr Oncol Rep 2020;22(8):85.

9. Grabher BJ. Breast cancer: evaluating tumor estrogen receptor status with molecular imaging to increase response to therapy and improve patient outcomes. J Nucl Med Technol 2020;48(3):191–201.

10. van Kruchten M, de Vries EGE, Brown M, et al. PET imaging of oestrogen receptors in patients with breast cancer. Lancet Oncol 2013;14(11):e465–75.

11. Yoo J, Dence CS, Sharp TL, et al. Synthesis of an estrogen receptor beta-selective radioligand: 5-[18F]fluoro-(2R,3S)-2,3-bis(4-hydroxyphenyl)pentanenitrile and comparison of in vivo distribution with 16alpha-[18F]fluoro-17beta-estradiol. J Med Chem 2005;48(20):6366–78.

12. Chae SY, Ahn SH, Kim SB, et al. Diagnostic accuracy and safety of 16α-[18F]fluoro-17β-oestradiol PET-CT for the assessment of oestrogen receptor status in recurrent or metastatic lesions in patients with breast cancer: a prospective cohort study. Lancet Oncol 2019;20(4):546–55.

13. Chae SY, Kim SB, Ahn SH, et al. A randomized feasibility study of 18F-Fluoroestradiol PET to predict pathologic response to neoadjuvant therapy in estrogen receptor-rich postmenopausal breast cancer. J Nucl Med 2017;58(4):563–8.

14. Gemignani ML, Patil S, Seshan VE, et al. Feasibility and predictability of perioperative PET and estrogen receptor ligand in patients with invasive breast cancer. J Nucl Med 2013;54(10):1697–702.

15. FDA label cerianna. Available at: https://www.accessdata.fda.gov/drugsatfda_docs/label/2020/212155s000lbl.pdf. Accessed March 10, 2022.

16. Mankoff DA, Peterson LM, Tewson TJ, et al. [18F]Fluoroestradiol radiation dosimetry in human PET studies. J Nucl Med 2001;42(4):679.

17. Mankoff DA, Clark AS. PET oestrogen receptor imaging: ready for the clinic? Lancet Oncol 2019;20(4):467–9.

18. Linden HM, Kurland BF, Peterson LM, et al. Fluoroestradiol positron emission tomography reveals differences in pharmacodynamics of aromatase inhibitors, tamoxifen, and fulvestrant in patients with metastatic breast cancer. Clin Cancer Res 2011;17(14):4799–805.

19. Evangelista L, Dieci MV, Guarneri V, Conte PF. 18F-Fluoroestradiol positron emission tomography in breast cancer patients: systematic review of the literature & meta-analysis. Curr Radiopharm 2016;9(3):244–57.

20. Kurland BF, Wiggins JR, Coche A, et al. Whole-body characterization of estrogen receptor status in metastatic breast cancer with 16α-18F-Fluoro-17β-Estradiol positron emission tomography: meta-analysis and recommendations for integration into clinical applications. Oncologist 2020;25(10):835–44.

21. Ivanidze J, Subramanian K, Youn T, et al. Utility of [18F]-fluoroestradiol (FES) PET/CT with dedicated brain acquisition in differentiating brain metastases from post-treatment change in estrogen receptor-positive breast cancer. Neurooncol Adv 2021;3(1):vdab178.

22. Katzenellenbogen JA. The quest for improving the management of breast cancer by functional imaging: The discovery and development of 16α-[18F]fluoroestradiol (FES), a PET radiotracer for the estrogen receptor, a historical review. Nucl Med Biol 2021;92:24–37.

23. Mortimer JE, Dehdashti F, Siegel BA, et al. Metabolic flare: indicator of hormone responsiveness in advanced breast cancer. J Clin Oncol 2001;19(11):2797–803.

24. Linden HM, Stekhova SA, Link JM, et al. Quantitative fluoroestradiol positron emission tomography imaging predicts response to endocrine treatment in breast cancer. J Clin Oncol 2006;24(18):2793–9.

25. Dehdashti F, Mortimer JE, Trinkaus K, et al. PET-based estradiol challenge as a predictive biomarker of response to endocrine therapy in women with estrogen-receptor-positive breast cancer. Breast Cancer Res Treat 2009;113(3):509–17.

26. Kurland BF, Peterson LM, Lee JH, et al. Estrogen receptor binding (18F-FES PET) and glycolytic activity (18F-FDG PET) predict progression-free survival on endocrine therapy in patients with ER+ breast cancer. Clin Cancer Res 2017;23(2):407–15.

27. van Kruchten M, de Vries EG, Glaudemans AW, et al. Measuring residual estrogen receptor availability during fulvestrant therapy in patients with metastatic breast cancer. Cancer Discov 2015;5(1):72–81.

28. Johnston SRD, Harbeck N, Hegg R, et al. Abemaciclib combined with endocrine therapy for the adjuvant treatment of HR+, HER2−, node-positive, high-risk, early breast cancer (monarchE). J Clin Oncol 2020. https://doi.org/10.1200/JCO.20.02514.

29. Boers J, Venema CM, de Vries EFJ, et al. Molecular imaging to identify patients with metastatic breast cancer who benefit from endocrine treatment combined with cyclin-dependent kinase inhibition. Eur J Cancer Oxf Engl 1990 2020;126:11–20.

30. Peterson LM, Kurland BF, Yan F, et al. 18F-Fluoroestradiol PET imaging in a phase II trial of vorinostat to restore endocrine sensitivity in ER+/HER2- metastatic breast cancer. J Nucl Med 2021;62(2):184–90.

31. Wang Y, Ayres KL, Goldman DA, et al. 18F-Fluoroestradiol PET/CT measurement of estrogen receptor suppression during a phase I trial of the novel estrogen receptor-targeted therapeutic GDC-0810: using an imaging biomarker to guide drug dosage in subsequent trials. Clin Cancer Res 2017;23(12):3053–60.

32. van Kruchten M, Glaudemans AWJM, de Vries EFJ, et al. PET imaging of estrogen receptors as a diagnostic tool for breast cancer patients presenting with a clinical dilemma. J Nucl Med 2012;53(2):182–90.

33. Sun Y, Yang Z, Zhang Y, et al. The preliminary study of 16α-[18F]fluoroestradiol PET/CT in assisting the individualized treatment decisions of breast cancer patients. PLoS One 2015;10(1):e0116341.

34. Venema C, de Vries E, Glaudemans A, et al. 18F-FES PET has added value in staging and therapy decision making in patients with disseminated lobular breast cancer. Clin Nucl Med 2017;42(8):612–4.

35. Ulaner GA, Jhaveri K, Chandarlapaty S, et al. Head-to-head evaluation of 18F-FES and 18F-FDG PET/CT in metastatic invasive lobular breast cancer. J Nucl Med 2021;62(3):326–31.

36. Boers J, Loudini N, de Haas RJ, et al. Analyzing the estrogen receptor status of liver metastases with [18F]-FES-PET in patients with breast cancer. Diagn Basel Switz 2021;11(11). 2019.

37. Koleva-Kolarova RG, Greuter MJW, Feenstra TL, et al. Molecular imaging with positron emission tomography and computed tomography (PET/CT) for selecting first-line targeted treatment in metastatic breast cancer: a cost-effectiveness study. Oncotarget 2018;9(28):19836–46.

38. Peterson LM, Kurland BF, Link JM, et al. Factors influencing the uptake of 18F-fluoroestradiol in patients with estrogen receptor positive breast cancer. Nucl Med Biol 2011;38(7):969–78.

39. Hathi DK, Li W, Seo Y, et al. Evaluation of primary breast cancers using dedicated breast PET and whole-body PET. Sci Rep 2020;10(1):21930.

40. Jones EF, Ray KM, Li W, et al. Initial experience of dedicated breast PET imaging of ER+ breast cancers using [F-18]fluoroestradiol. NPJ Breast Cancer 2019; 5(1):1–6.

41. Miyake KK, Kataoka M, Ishimori T, et al. A proposed dedicated breast pet lexicon: standardization of description and reporting of radiotracer uptake in the breast. Diagn Basel Switz 2021;11(7):1267.

42. Liao GJ, Clark AS, Schubert EK, et al. 18F-Fluoroestradiol PET: current status and potential future clinical applications. J Nucl Med 2016;57(8):1269–75.

43. van Kruchten M, Glaudemans AWJM, de Vries EFJ, et al. Positron emission tomography of tumour [(18)F]fluoroestradiol uptake in patients with acquired hormone-resistant metastatic breast cancer prior to oestradiol therapy. Eur J Nucl Med Mol Imaging 2015;42(11):1674–81.

44. Ulaner G. 18F-Fluoroestradiol (FES) PET/CT Compared to standard-of-care imaging in patients with breast cancer. clinicaltrials.gov. 2022. Available at: https://clinicaltrials.gov/ct2/show/NCT04883814. Accessed March 3, 2022.

45. Gennari A, Brain E, Nanni O, et al. 114P - Molecular imaging with 18F-fluoroestradiol (18F-FES) to assess intra-patient heterogeneity in metastatic breast cancer (MBC): a European TRANSCAN program. Annals of Oncology 2017;28(suppl_5): v22-v42. doi:10.1093/annonc/mdx363.030

5-Aminolevulinic Acid Imaging of Malignant Glioma

Guan Li, BS, Adrian Rodrigues, BA, Lily Kim, MD, Cesar Garcia, BS, Shruti Jain, PhD, Michael Zhang, MD, Melanie Hayden-Gephart, MAS, MD*

KEYWORDS

- 5-Aminolevulinic acid • 5-ALA • Glioma • Fluorescence-guided surgery
- Brain tumor resection

KEY POINTS

- Exogenous dosing of 5-aminolevulinic acid (5-ALA) can be used to differentially visualize high-grade glioma from normal brain under fluorescence-guided surgery (FGS).
- The use of 5-ALA FGS has been shown to improve the extent of resection; extent of resection is correlated with improved 6-month progression free survival and overall survival in patients with high-grade glioma.
- The intensity of fluorescence is largely determined by tumor characteristics such as grade, density, and mutational status.
- Limitations of 5-ALA FGS include administration window, decreased sensitivity around the infiltrating tumor border, and poor visualization of low-grade gliomas.
- Emerging technologies such as photodynamic therapy, intraoperative ultrasound, intraoperative MRI, and simulated Raman histology may offer additional advantages in combination with 5-ALA FGS.

 Video content accompanies this article at http://www.surgonc.theclinics.com.

INTRODUCTION

High-grade gliomas (HGGs) are the most common primary malignant brain tumors in adults.[1] HGGs have an overall poor prognosis with a median survival of 15 months.[2] In lower risk patients with surgically accessible tumors, maximal safe tumor resection followed by adjuvant chemoradiotherapy is the standard of care.[3–6] In patients who qualify for tumor resection (low operative risk), extent of resection (EOR) studies

Department of Neurosurgery, Stanford School of Medicine, 300 Pasteur Drive, Stanford, CA 94305, USA
* Corresponding author.
E-mail address: mghayden@stanford.edu

Surg Oncol Clin N Am 31 (2022) 581–593
https://doi.org/10.1016/j.soc.2022.06.002

Abbreviations	
5-ALA	5-aminolevulinic acid
CRET	Complete Resection of Enhanced Tissue
CR	Complete Resection
EOR	Extent of Resection
FGS	Fluorescence-Guided Surgery
GTR	Gross Total Resection
OS	Overall Survival
PFS	Progression-Free Survival

have associated maximal safe tumor resection with modest benefits in quality of life, progression-free survival (PFS), and overall survival (OS), so long as the patient does not suffer from a significant decline in neurologic or medical function.[7–12] The infiltrative nature of gliomas into the surrounding brain parenchyma makes it difficult during surgery to delineate tumor versus normal brain tissue.[3] Following Food and Drug Administration (FDA) approval in 2017, fluorescence-guided surgery (FGS) of HGG using 5-aminolevulinic acid (5-ALA) has become widely adopted.[13] Exogenous 5-ALA selectively accumulates in HGG tissue, allowing for improved intraoperative visualization with a fluorescence microscope, which when combined with expert neurosurgical knowledge of brain anatomy, allows for maximal safe tumor resection.[13] This review provides an overview of the use of 5-ALA in HGG resection, its benefits, limitations, and future applications.

BIOCHEMISTRY OF 5-AMINOLEVULINIC ACID

5-ALA (molecular weight 131.13 g/mol) is an endogenous, nonfluorescent intermediate in the heme biosynthesis pathway (**Fig. 1**).[14] It is naturally synthesized from the condensation of glycine and succinyl-coenzyme A by 5-ALA synthase and is subsequently converted to protoporphyrin IX (PpIX), a fluorescent intermediate product of heme metabolism.[14,15] In HGG, normal regulation of the 5-ALA-PpIX metabolic pathway is disrupted, and large amounts of PpIX accumulate within the tumor cells.[16] Although the exact mechanism for why malignant cells exhibit preferential intracellular accumulation of PpIX remains unclear, several hypotheses have been proposed including disruptions in the regulation and turnover of PpIX.[16] Exogenous application of 5-ALA leads to the accumulation of PpIX; when excited with blue light, the emitting red-violet light (fluorescence) can be detected with a properly equipped operative microscope and allow for 5-ALA FGS.[13]

5-Aminolevulinic Acid Protocol

The FDA standard protocol calls for oral administration of 5-ALA 3 hours before the induction of anesthesia, dosed at 20 mg/kg dissolved in 50 mL of water.[13,17,18] The timing of administration may need to be adjusted based on logistical challenges and complexity of the surgical approach to the tumor. During tumor resection, conventional white light is switched to blue light (λ = 400–410 nm) for tissue excitation. PpIX-induced tumor fluorescence (approx. 635 nm)[19,20] is then visualized using an operative microscope with a red-violet light filter (**Fig. 2**, Video 1).[19,20] After the surgery, patients are monitored and protected from strong light sources for 48 hours to prevent skin photosensitivity.[21–23]

Complications from use of 5-ALA consist of drug side effects and neurologic injury from surgical excision of eloquent cortex.[24] 5-ALA administration has been proven to

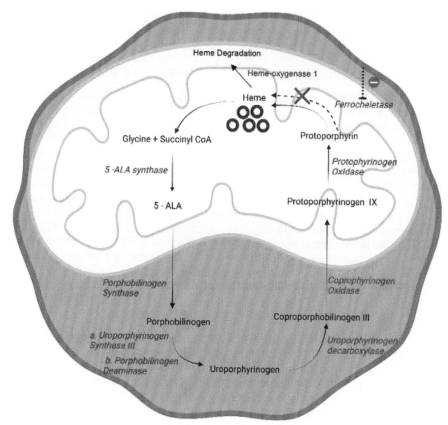

Fig. 1. Biochemical pathway of 5-ALA metabolism.

be safe with minimal complications.[17,25–31] PpIX has photosensitization properties, but phototoxic events are rarely observed.[32–34] Hypotension after 5-ALA administration was most associated with a history of hypertension and use of antihypertensive therapy (odds ratio = 17.7).[23] Mild elevation of liver enzymes with no other signs of

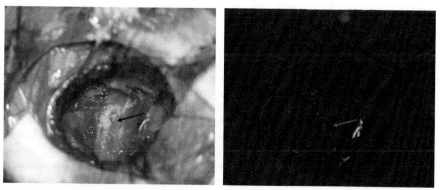

Fig. 2. Intraoperative images during glioma surgery in white light (*left*) and fluorescence mode (*right*). Tumor core indicated by the arrows.

hepatic disorder has also been reported.[17,25] 5-ALA is contraindicated in patients with hypersensitivity to 5-ALA hydrochloride or porphyrins, acute or chronic types of porphyria, or pregnancy.[35]

BENEFITS OF 5-AMINOLEVULINIC ACID FLUORESCENCE-GUIDED SURGERY

The use of 5-ALA FGS has been shown to improve the EOR in HGG and improve clinical outcomes.[17,25,36-40] EOR studies have reported gross total resection of malignant gliomas ranging from 47.4% to 96% of cases in the 5-ALA group compared with 22.9% to 51.4% of cases in the conventional white light group.[10,21,24,25,38,39,41-45] As a result of this increased EOR, patients are also reported to have higher 6-month PFS and OS.[25,39,40] In a recent single-center retrospective cohort study (N = 343), the authors found that the use of 5-ALA FGS in glioblastoma resection was associated with improved OS (17.47 vs 10.63 months, $P < .0001$), fewer new focal neurologic deficits (23.3% vs 44.9%, $P < .0001$), and larger EOR (gross total resection 47.4% vs 22.9%, $P < .0001$).[39] In a randomized, controlled, multicenter phase III trial (N = 322), the authors reported that patients in the 5-ALA FGS group had a longer 6-month progression free survival than those in the white light group (41.0% vs 21.1% $P = .0003$, Z test).[25] A summary of studies examining the impact of 5-ALA FGS on EOR, PFS, and OS is presented in **Table 1**.

FACTORS AFFECTING 5-AMINOLEVULINIC ACID FLUORESCENCE

Several factors affect the efficacy of 5-ALA FGS, such as timing of administration, tumor grade, tumor necrosis, tumor density, and molecular features. In current clinical practice, it is advised to administer 5-ALA at a dose of 20 mg/kg of body weight at 3 hours before induction with anesthesia.[25,47,48] The recommendation was based on findings in earlier studies where peak PpIX fluorescence was 6 hours after administration.[49] However, more recent studies have shown that PpIX fluorescence and tumor PpIX concentration peaks between 7 and 8 hours after 5-ALA administration.[49] This observation is suggestive that 5-ALA can be administered at earlier time points (4–5 hours) before planned tumor resection.[49]

Tumor grade affects the amount of intracellular PpIX accumulation and overall fluorescence. Clinical guidelines recommend the use of 5-ALA FGS for HGG but not for low-grade glioma.[13,50-53] It is well known that the intracellular accumulation of PpIX in low-grade gliomas (LGG) is generally insufficient to elicit a positive fluorescent signal that can be detected during surgery.[50-53] Several clinical studies have failed to show improved outcomes for patients with LGG after receiving 5-ALA FGS.[50-53] However, it has been shown that areas of fluorescence within LGG can correlate with anaplastic foci, including overlap with areas of contrast enhancement on MRI or positive signal in positron emission tomography.[53,54] If methods to detect fluorescence improve, it may be possible to use 5-ALA FGS to identify active areas of tumor growth in LGGs. For example, one study used a dual detection system with both FGS to detect fluorescence intensity and a handheld spectroscopic probe to measure PpIX intracellular concentration.[52] The dual detection system allowed the authors to measure significant increases in PpIX concentration even in nonfluorescent LGG tissue when compared with a cutoff value of 0.005 μg/mL used to distinguish between nontumor and tumor tissue (generated from a receiver operating characteristic curve analysis).[55]

Tumor heterogeneity, including necrosis (a defining characteristic of glioblastoma), will influence PpIX accumulation and fluorescence. It has been shown that 5-ALA fluorescence is maximal within the tumor core and can be visualized with a bright red coloration.[13,56-58] In contrast, the tumor periphery or infiltrating edge will possess

Table 1
Summary of studies examining the impact of 5-ALA FGS on EOR, PFS, and OS

	Study Type	Number of Patients	EOR	PFS	OS
Stummer et al,[25] 2006	Randomized controlled multicenter phase III trial	N = 270	5-ALA: 65% CRET WL: 36% CRET P<.0001	6-mo PFS: 5-ALA: 41.0% WL: 21.1% P = .0003	Median OS: 5-ALA 15.2 mo WL: 13.5 mo P = .1
Stummer et al,[24] 2011	Randomized controlled multicenter phase III trial	N = 349	5-ALA: 63.6% CRET WL: 37.6 CRET P<.0001	6-mo PFS: 5-ALA: 35.2% WL: 21.8% P = .004	Median OS: 5-ALA: 14.3 mo WL: 13.7 mo P = .917
Eljamel,[41] 2015	Meta-analyses	N = 565	5-ALA: 75.4% GTR	Mean PFS: 8.1 mo	Difference in OS vs WL: 6.2 mo
Cordova et al,[42] 2016	Prospective	N = 30	5-ALA–Median EOR: 94.8%, 30% CRET 53.3% GTR	6-mo PFS: 45%	6-mo OS: 81%
Schucht et al,[38] 2012	Prospective	N = 53	5-ALA: 96% GTR 89% CRET	N/A	N/A
Idoate et al,[43] 2013	Prospective	N = 30	5-ALA: EOR>98% 83.3% GTR	N/A	N/A
Kim et al,[44] 2014	Prospective	N = 80	Mean EOR: 5-ALA 97.0% WL: 84.7% 5-ALA: 80% CRET WL: 43% CRET P = .002	Median PFS: 5-ALA 18.0 mo WL: 6.0 mo P = .001	Median OS: 5-ALA: 24.0 mo WL: 14.0 mo P = .045
Teixidor et al,[21] 2016	Prospective	N = 85	5-ALA: 53.9% CR	6 mo PFS: 58% Median PFS: 6.9 mo	6-mo OS: 78.4% Median OS: 14.2 mo

(continued on next page)

Table 1
(continued)

	Study Type	Number of Patients	EOR	PFS	OS
Slotty et al,[45] 2013	Multicentric retrospective	N = 253	5-ALA 48.5% CR WL: 21.4% −27.2% CR P<.01	N/A	N/A
Picart et al,[46] 2017	Multicentric retrospective	N = 51	5-ALA: 67.3% GTR WL: 51.4% GTR P = .05	6-mo PFS: 5-ALA: 97% WL: 55% Median PFS: 5-ALA: 13.21 mo WL: 7.24 mo P = .03	6-mo OS: 5-ALA: 96% WL: 93% Median OS: 5-ALA: 25 mo WL: 12 mo P = .080
Baig Mirza et al,[39] 2021	Single center retrospective	N = 343	5-ALA: 47.4% GTR WL: 22.9% GTR	N/A	5-ALA: 17.47 mo WL: 10.63 mo

Abbreviations: 5-ALA FGS, 5-aminolevulinic acid fluorescence-guided surgery; CR, complete resection; CRET, complete resection of enhanced tissue; EOR, extent of resection; GTR, gross total resection; OS, overall survival; PFS, progression-free survival; WL, white light.

less fluorescence as shown by a lighter, faint pink coloration.[13,56–58] One explanation is that PpIX better accumulates in regions of higher tumor density, such as the core, and will decrease in diffuse tumor regions such as the invasive edge.[13,56–59]

Other features affecting 5-ALA fluorescence include photobleaching and tumor molecular features. It has been shown that PpIX fluorescence will decay over time, and the rate of decay depends on the initial light source used from the microscope to visualize the signal.[60] Two studies found that decay rate could decrease to 36% when exposed to 12.4 ± 8.6 J/cm^2 irradiance with 8 mW/cm^2 microscope light intensity.[58,60] With prolonged surgical times, it becomes more difficult to detect tumor tissue at the invasive front or in tumor areas with less fluorescence.

5-ALA is often administered before biopsy and molecular characterization of the tumor but molecular features do play a role in PpIX accumulation. Although molecular grading systems have recently changed,[61] in a retrospective study of World Health Organization grade II – IV gliomas, intraoperative fluorescence was significantly higher for IDH1/2 WT status compared with IDH1/2 mutant (n = 104; $P < .01$).[62] One proposed mechanism for the observed difference was that IDH1/2 mutant HGG expressed higher levels of ferrochelatase and heme-oxygenase 1, which metabolized PpIX and decreased the intracellular concentration.[16,62,63]

In summary, timing of 5-ALA administration, tumor grade, tumor necrosis, tumor density, and molecular features should be considered in FGS protocols.

USE OF 5-AMINOLEVULINIC ACID AS DUAL IMAGING AND PHOTODYNAMIC THERAPY

Apart from its use as a fluorescent marker to demarcate tumor boundaries, studies are currently underway to use 5-ALA in photodynamic therapy (PDT), wherein preferential accumulation of PpIX in tumor cells allows for therapeutic targeting. The surgical workflow would be to first use the excitatory wavelength for 5-ALA tumor resection, and then apply PDT at a different wavelength (635 nm) to the resection cavity.[19,20,64–66] On activation, the photosensitizer would produce reactive oxygen species, inducing cytotoxicity, local ischemia by damaging neoplastic vessels, and immune responses.[64–67] Several limitations of PDT with 5-ALA include unequal uptake of 5-ALA across tumor cells, which can result in therapy resistance in certain cell populations. Technical limitations include shallow depths of light penetration, where the light source must be placed near the photosensitizer, and long exposure times to generate a therapeutic effect.[23] If successful, this approach would allow surgeons to target infiltrating residual tumor cells with PDT.

This dual functionality is currently under clinical trial. In a phase 1 clinical trial called Intraoperative Photodynamic Therapy of Glioblastoma, intraoperative PDT is applied to the resection cavity following FGS with 5-ALA.[68] In a phase 1 to 2 study (N = 23) where a hematoporphyrin derivative was used for FGS and PDT, no direct complications resulted from PDT.[69] In a similar study of FGS and PDT in patients with recurrent HGG (n = 20), the only adverse effect reported was one infection, and a median PFS of 6 months (95% CI 4.8–7.2 mos) but the PFS was not different than historical controls.[67] PDT has been FDA approved in the treatment of other cancers such as Barrett's esophagus and obstructing esophageal carcinoma[70]; further clinical trials are needed to assess the efficacy of 5-ALA PDT in HGG.[64]

OPTIMIZATION AND DEVELOPING ALTERNATIVES TO 5-AMINOLEVULINIC ACID

Additional fluorescent compounds are under active study, including EGFR-targeted fluorophore-labelled antibody (ABY-029), a fluorescent antibiotic (demeclocycline), and a protease-activated fluorescent probe (LUM015).[3,71–73] Intraoperative tumor visualization can also be affected by photobleaching, and there is some evidence that PpIX is more susceptible to this phenomenon than other fluorophores, including the commonly used Alexa Fluor agents.[74] Surgical loupe laser excitation has been trialed to enhance the degree of intraoperative fluorescence.[75] Others are investigating methods to quantitatively detect PpIX levels with fiber-optic probes and intraoperative spectroscopy.[76,77]

Additional methods currently used to assist in improving EOR include intraoperative ultrasound (ioUS), intraoperative MRI (iMRI), and simulated Raman histology (SRH). ioUS, relying on different echogenicity patterns between normal brain and tumor, offers fast, real-time, inexpensive imaging to detect residual tumor and improve EOR.[78,79] However, accurate interpretation requires significant user experience, and tumor and normal brain structures may share acoustic gradients and produce similar echoic patterns. iMRI, more frequently used in LGG, requires interruption of surgery to scan the patient, the cost of building operating room-adjacent MRI suites, and the use of high-field (>1T) scanners. SRH by contrast is an ex vivo technique to aid in surgical diagnosis and determine the extent of infiltrating tumor cells in surgical margins.[80–83] Indeed, a synergistic approach between intraoperative imaging methods may confer the greatest surgical benefit.[84] One study found that the use of high-field iMRI with 5-ALA increased the EOR in HGGs adjacent to eloquent areas from 61.7% to 100%.[85] Additional studies are needed to determine the future use of molecular fluorophores, SRH, iMRI, and/or ioUS to optimize the maximal safe resection of HGG.

SUMMARY

The introduction of 5-ALA FGS in HGG surgery has provided surgeons with a valuable tool to improve EOR. 5-ALA FGS is not effective across all glioma subtypes due to differences in tumor density and metabolism. Advances in the use of 5-ALA and novel intraoperative imaging adjuncts may help overcome current limitations.

CLINICS CARE POINTS

- 5-aminolevulinic acid (5-ALA) fluorescence-guided surgery is an effective method to improve intraoperative HGG visualization.
- 5-ALA has a therapeutic dosing window for tumor resection between 4 and 8 hours.
- Expert surgical knowledge of neuroanatomy is required to avoid postoperative neurologic deficits.
- Side effects include photosensitivity (avoid strong light sources for 48 hours), hypotension, and mild disruption of liver function.
- 5-ALA is contraindicated in patients with hypersensitivity to 5-ALA hydrochloride or porphyrins, acute or chronic types of porphyria, or pregnancy.

DISCLOSURE

The authors have nothing to disclose.

SUPPLEMENTARY DATA

Supplementary data related to this article can be found online at https://doi.org/10.1016/j.soc.2022.06.002.

REFERENCES

1. Ostrom QT, Gittleman H, Truitt G, et al. CBTRUS Statistical Report: Primary brain and Other Central Nervous system tumors diagnosed in the United States in 2011–2015. Neuro-Oncology 2018;iv1–86.
2. Fernandes C, Costa A, Osório L, et al. Current Standards of care in glioblastoma therapy. In: De Vleeschouwer S, editor. Glioblastoma [Internet]. Brisbane (AU): Codon Publications; 2017. Chapter 11. Available at: Https://Www.Ncbi.Nlm.Nih.-Gov/Books/NBK469987/Doi: 10.15586/Codon.Glioblastoma.2017.Ch11.
3. Sun R, Cuthbert H, Watts C. Fluorescence-Guided surgery in the surgical treatment of gliomas: Past, present and future. Cancers (Basel) 2021;13(14):3508.
4. Medikonda R, Dunn G, Rahman M, et al. A review of glioblastoma immunotherapy. J Neurooncol 2021;151(1):41–53.
5. Stupp R, Mason WP, van den Bent MJ, et al. Radiotherapy plus Concomitant and adjuvant Temozolomide for glioblastoma. N Engl J Med 2005;352(10):987–96.
6. Di Carlo DT, Cagnazzo F, Benedetto N, et al. Multiple high-grade gliomas: epidemiology, management, and outcome. A systematic review and meta-analysis. Neurosurg Rev 2019;42(2):263–75.
7. D'Amico RS, Englander ZK, Canoll P, et al. Extent of resection in glioma–A review of the Cutting Edge. World Neurosurg 2017;103:538–49.
8. Khatri D, Das KK, Gosal JS, et al. Surgery in high-grade Insular tumors: Oncological and Seizure outcomes from 41 consecutive patients. Asian J Neurosurg 2020;15(3):537–44.
9. Khatri D, Jaiswal A, Das K, et al. Health-related quality of life after surgery in supratentorial gliomas. Neurol India 2019;67(2):467.
10. Picart T, Berhouma M, Dumot C, et al. Optimization of high-grade glioma resection using 5-ALA fluorescence-guided surgery: a literature review and practical recommendations from the neuro-oncology club of the French society of neurosurgery. Neurochirurgie 2019;65(4):164–77.
11. Brown TJ, Brennan MC, Li M, et al. Association of the extent of resection with survival in glioblastoma: a systematic review and meta-analysis. JAMA Oncol 2016;2(11):1460.
12. Rahman M, Abbatematteo J, De Leo EK, et al. The effects of new or worsened postoperative neurological deficits on survival of patients with glioblastoma. J Neurosurg 2017;127(1):123–31.
13. Dadario NB, Khatri D, Reichman N, et al. 5-Aminolevulinic acid–Shedding Light on where to Focus. World Neurosurg 2021;150:9–16.
14. Layer G, Reichelt J, Jahn D, et al. Structure and function of enzymes in heme biosynthesis. Protein Sci 2010;19(6):1137–61.
15. Stummer W, Stocker S, Novotny A, et al. In vitro and in vivo porphyrin accumulation by C6 glioma cells after exposure to 5-aminolevulinic acid. J Photochem Photobiol B: Biol 1998;45(2–3):160–9.
16. Kim JE, Cho HR, Xu WJ, et al. Mechanism for enhanced 5-aminolevulinic acid fluorescence in isocitrate dehydrogenase 1 mutant malignant gliomas. Oncotarget 2015;6(24):20266–77.
17. Stummer W, Novotny A, Stepp H, et al. Fluorescence-guided resection of glioblastoma multiforme utilizing 5-ALA-induced porphyrins: a prospective study in 52 consecutive patients. J Neurosurg 2000;93(6):1003–13.
18. Walter S, Susanne S, Simon W, et al. Intraoperative detection of malignant gliomas by 5-aminolevulinic acid-induced porphyrin fluorescence. Neurosurgery 1998;42(3):518–26.

19. Wei L, Roberts DW, Sanai N, et al. Visualization technologies for 5-ALA-based fluorescence-guided surgeries. J Neurooncol 2019;141(3):495–505.

20. Stummer W, Stepp H, Wiestler OD, et al. Randomized, prospective Double-Blinded study Comparing 3 Different Doses of 5-aminolevulinic acid for fluorescence-guided resections of malignant gliomas. Neurosurgery 2017;81(2):230–9.

21. Teixidor P, Arráez MÁ, Villalba G, et al. Safety and Efficacy of 5-aminolevulinic acid for high Grade glioma in Usual clinical practice: a prospective cohort study. PLoS ONE 2016;11(2):e0149244.

22. Webber J, Kessel D, Fromm D. Plasma levels of protoporphyrin IX in humans after oral administration of 5-aminolevulinic acid. J Photochem Photobiol B: Biol 1997; 37(1–2):151–3.

23. Chung IWH, Eljamel S. Risk factors for developing oral 5-aminolevulenic acid-induced side effects in patients undergoing fluorescence guided resection. Photodiagnosis Photodynamic Ther 2013;10(4):362–7.

24. Stummer W, Tonn JC, Mehdorn HM, et al. Counterbalancing risks and gains from extended resections in malignant glioma surgery: a supplemental analysis from the randomized 5-aminolevulinic acid glioma resection study: clinical article. JNS 2011;114(3):613–23.

25. Stummer W, Pichlmeier U, Meinel T, et al. Fluorescence-guided surgery with 5-aminolevulinic acid for resection of malignant glioma: a randomised controlled multicentre phase III trial. The Lancet Oncol 2006;7(5):392–401.

26. Dalton JT, Yates CR, Yin D, et al. Clinical Pharmacokinetics of 5-aminolevulinic acid in healthy Volunteers and patients at high Risk for recurrent bladder cancer. J Pharmacol Exp Ther 2002;301(2):507–12.

27. Peng Q, Warloe T, Berg K, et al. 5-Aminolevulinic acid-based photodynamic therapy: clinical research and future challenges. Cancer 1997;79(12):2282–308.

28. Eljamel MS. Photodynamic assisted surgical resection and treatment of malignant brain tumours technique, technology and clinical application. Photodiagnosis Photodynamic Ther 2004;1(1):93–8.

29. Eljamel MS. Fluorescence image-guided surgery of brain tumors: Explained step-by-step. Photodiagnosis Photodynamic Ther 2008;5(4):260–3.

30. Zilidis G, Aziz F, Telara S, et al. Fluorescence image-guided surgery and repetitive Photodynamic Therapy in brain metastatic malignant melanoma. Photodiagnosis Photodynamic Ther 2008;5(4):264–6.

31. Aziz F, Telara S, Moseley H, et al. Photodynamic therapy adjuvant to surgery in metastatic carcinoma in brain. Photodiagnosis Photodynamic Ther 2009;6(3–4): 227–30.

32. Hickmann AK, Nadji-Ohl M, Hopf NJ. Feasibility of fluorescence-guided resection of recurrent gliomas using five-aminolevulinic acid: retrospective analysis of surgical and neurological outcome in 58 patients. J Neurooncol 2015;122(1):151–60.

33. Panciani PP, Fontanella M, Schatlo B, et al. Fluorescence and image guided resection in high grade glioma. Clin Neurol Neurosurg 2012;114(1):37–41.

34. Aldave G, Tejada S, Pay E, et al. Prognostic value of residual Fluorescent tissue in glioblastoma patients after Gross Total resection in 5-aminolevulinic acid-guided surgery. Neurosurgery 2013;72(6):915–21.

35. European medicines Agency. Available at: https://Www.Ema.Europa.Eu/En/Documents/Scientific-Discussion/Gliolan-Epar-Scientific-Discussion_en.Pdf. Accessed January 19, 2022.

36. McGirt MJ, Chaichana KL, Gathinji M, et al. Independent association of extent of resection with survival in patients with malignant brain astrocytoma: clinical article. JNS 2009;110(1):156–62.

37. Schucht P, Seidel K, Beck J, et al. Intraoperative monopolar mapping during 5-ALA–guided resections of glioblastomas adjacent to motor eloquent areas: evaluation of resection rates and neurological outcome. FOC 2014;37(6):E16.

38. Schucht P, Beck J, Abu-Isa J, et al. Gross Total resection rates in Contemporary glioblastoma surgery. Neurosurgery 2012;71(5):927–36.

39. Baig Mirza A, Christodoulides I, Lavrador JP, et al. 5-Aminolevulinic acid-guided resection improves the overall survival of patients with glioblastoma—a comparative cohort study of 343 patients. Neuro-Oncology Adv 2021;3(1):vdab047.

40. Vogelbaum MA, Jost S, Aghi MK, et al. Application of Novel Response/Progression Measures for Surgically delivered therapies for gliomas. Neurosurgery 2012; 70(1):234–44.

41. Eljamel S. 5-ALA fluorescence image guided resection of glioblastoma multiforme: a meta-analysis of the literature. IJMS 2015;16(12):10443–56.

42. Cordova JS, Gurbani SS, Holder CA, et al. Semi-automated Volumetric and Morphological Assessment of glioblastoma resection with fluorescence-guided surgery. Mol Imaging Biol 2016;18(3):454–62.

43. Idoate MA, Díez Valle R, Echeveste J, et al. Pathological characterization of the glioblastoma border as shown during surgery using 5-aminolevulinic acid-induced fluorescence: Pathology of glioblastoma border. Neuropathology 2011; 31(6):575–82.

44. Kim SK, Choi SH, Kim YH, et al. Impact of fluorescence-guided surgery on the improvement of clinical outcomes in glioblastoma patients. Neuro-Oncology Pract 2014;1(3):81–5.

45. Slotty PJ, Siantidis B, Beez T, et al. The impact of improved treatment strategies on overall survival in glioblastoma patients. Acta Neurochir 2013;155(6):959–63.

46. Picart T, Armoiry X, Berthiller J, et al. Is fluorescence-guided surgery with 5-ala in eloquent areas for malignant gliomas a reasonable and useful technique? Neurochirurgie 2017 Jun;63(3):189–96.

47. Maragkos GA, Schüpper AJ, Lakomkin N, et al. Fluorescence-Guided high-grade glioma surgery More than Four Hours after 5-aminolevulinic acid administration. Front Neurol 2021;12:644804.

48. Schupper AJ, Rao M, Mohammadi N, et al. Fluorescence-Guided surgery: a review on Timing and Use in brain tumor surgery. Front Neurol 2021;12:682151.

49. Kaneko S, Suero Molina E, Ewelt C, et al. Fluorescence-Based Measurement of Real-Time Kinetics of protoporphyrin IX after 5-aminolevulinic acid administration in human in Situ malignant gliomas. Neurosurgery 2019;85(4):E739–46.

50. Hervey-Jumper SL, Berger MS. Maximizing safe resection of low- and high-grade glioma. J Neurooncol 2016;130(2):269–82.

51. Lau D, Hervey-Jumper SL, Chang S, et al. A prospective Phase II clinical trial of 5-aminolevulinic acid to assess the correlation of intraoperative fluorescence intensity and degree of histologic cellularity during resection of high-grade gliomas. JNS 2016;124(5):1300–9.

52. Widhalm G, Olson J, Weller J, et al. The value of visible 5-ALA fluorescence and quantitative protoporphyrin IX analysis for improved surgery of suspected low-grade gliomas. J Neurosurg 2020;133(1):79–88.

53. Hendricks BK, Sanai N, Stummer W. Fluorescence-guided surgery with aminolevulinic acid for low-grade gliomas. J Neurooncol 2019;141(1):13–8.

54. Widhalm G, Wolfsberger S, Minchev G, et al. 5-Aminolevulinic acid is a promising marker for detection of anaplastic foci in diffusely infiltrating gliomas with nonsignificant contrast enhancement. Cancer 2010;116(6):1545–52.

55. Widhalm G, Olson J, Weller J, et al. The value of visible 5-ALA fluorescence and quantitative protoporphyrin IX analysis for improved surgery of suspected low-grade gliomas. J Neurosurg Published Online May 2019;10:1–10.

56. Rampazzo E, Della Puppa A, Frasson C, et al. Phenotypic and functional characterization of Glioblastoma cancer stem cells identified through 5-aminolevulinic acid-assisted surgery [corrected]. J Neurooncol 2014;116(3):505–13.

57. Manini I, Caponnetto F, Dalla E, et al. Heterogeneity Matters: Different Regions of glioblastoma are Characterized by Distinctive tumor-Supporting Pathways. Cancers (Basel). 2020;12(10):E2960.

58. Stummer W, Stocker S, Wagner S, et al. Intraoperative detection of malignant gliomas by 5-aminolevulinic acid-induced porphyrin fluorescence. Neurosurgery 1998;42(3):518–25 [discussion: 525–6].

59. Johansson A, Palte G, Schnell O, et al. 5-Aminolevulinic acid-induced protoporphyrin IX levels in tissue of human malignant brain tumors: Photochemistry and Photobiology. Photochem Photobiol 2010;86(6):1373–8.

60. Belykh E, Miller EJ, Patel AA, et al. Optical characterization of Neurosurgical Operating Microscopes: quantitative fluorescence and Assessment of PpIX Photobleaching. Sci Rep 2018;8(1):12543.

61. Komori T. Grading of adult diffuse gliomas according to the 2021 WHO Classification of tumors of the Central Nervous system. Lab Invest 2022;102(2):126–33.

62. Ohba S, Murayama K, Kuwahara K, et al. The correlation of fluorescence of Protoporphyrinogen IX and Status of isocitrate dehydrogenase in gliomas. Neurosurgery 2020;87(2):408–17.

63. Schwake M, Günes D, Köchling M, et al. Kinetics of porphyrin fluorescence accumulation in pediatric brain tumor cells incubated in 5-aminolevulinic acid. Acta Neurochir 2014;156(6):1077–84.

64. Mahmoudi K, Garvey K, Bouras A, et al. 5-Aminolevulinic acid photodynamic therapy for the treatment of high-grade gliomas. J Neurooncol 2019;141(3):595–607.

65. Inoue K. 5-Aminolevulinic acid-mediated photodynamic therapy for bladder cancer. Int J Urol 2017;24(2):97–101.

66. Cramer SW, Chen CC. Photodynamic therapy for the treatment of glioblastoma. Front Surg 2020;6. Available at: https://www.frontiersin.org/article/10.3389/fsurg.2019.00081. Accessed January 18, 2022.

67. Schipmann S, Müther M, Stögbauer L, et al. Combination of ALA-induced fluorescence-guided resection and intraoperative open photodynamic therapy for recurrent glioblastoma: case series on a promising dual strategy for local tumor control. J Neurosurg 2020;134(2):426–36.

68. Dupont C, Vermandel M, Leroy HA, et al. INtraoperative photoDYnamic therapy for GliOblastomas (INDYGO): study Protocol for a phase I clinical trial. Neurosurgery 2019;84(6):E414–9.

69. Kaye AH, Morstyn G, Brownbill D. Adjuvant high-dose photoradiation therapy in the treatment of cerebral glioma: a phase 1-2 study. J Neurosurg 1987;67(4):500–5.

70. Biel M. Advances in photodynamic therapy for the treatment of head and neck cancers. Lasers Surg Med 2006;38(5):349–55.

71. ClinicalTrials.Gov. National Library of medicine (US) A phase 0 open Label, Single-Center clinical trial of ABY-029, an Anti-EGFR fluorescence Imaging Agent via Single Intravenous Injection to Subjects with recurrent glioma. [(Accessed January 23, 2021)]; Available at: Https://Clinicaltrials.Gov/Ct2/Show/NCT02901925.

72. ClinicalTrials.Gov. Bethesda (MD) National Library of medicine (US) Feasibility of the LUM Imaging system for in vivo and Ex vivo detection of cancer in Subjects with low Grade gliomas, glioblastomas, and cancer Metastases to the brain. [(Accessed January 23, 2021)]; Available at: Https://Clinicaltrials.Gov/Ct2/Show/NCT03717142.

73. ClinicalTrials.Gov. National Library of medicine (US) Demeclocycline fluorescence for intraoperative Delineation brain tumors. [(Accessed January 23, 2021)]; Available at: Https://Clinicaltrials.Gov/Ct2/Show/NCT02740933.

74. Valdes PA, Juvekar P, Agar NYR, et al. Quantitative Wide-Field Imaging Techniques for fluorescence guided neurosurgery. Front Surg 2019;6:31.

75. Kuroiwa T, Kajimoto Y, Furuse M, et al. A surgical loupe system for observing protoporphyrin IX fluorescence in high-grade gliomas after administering 5-aminolevulinic acid. Photodiagnosis Photodyn Ther 2013;10(4):379–81.

76. Richter JCO, Haj-Hosseini N, Hallbeck M, et al. Combination of hand-held probe and microscopy for fluorescence guided surgery in the brain tumor marginal zone. Photodiagnosis Photodyn Ther 2017;18:185–92.

77. Alston L, Mahieu-Williame L, Hebert M, et al. Spectral complexity of 5-ALA induced PpIX fluorescence in guided surgery: a clinical study towards the discrimination of healthy tissue and margin boundaries in high and low grade gliomas. Biomed Opt Express 2019;10(5):2478–92.

78. Trevisi G, Barbone P, Treglia G, et al. Reliability of intraoperative ultrasound in detecting tumor residual after brain diffuse glioma surgery: a systematic review and meta-analysis. Neurosurg Rev 2020;43(5):1221–33.

79. Mahboob S, McPhillips R, Qiu Z, et al. Intraoperative ultrasound-guided resection of gliomas: a meta-analysis and review of the literature. World Neurosurg 2016; 92:255–63.

80. Di L, Eichberg DG, Huang K, et al. Stimulated Raman histology for Rapid intraoperative Diagnosis of gliomas. World Neurosurg 2021;150:e135–43.

81. Orringer DA, Pandian B, Niknafs YS, et al. Rapid intraoperative histology of unprocessed surgical specimens via fibre-laser-based stimulated Raman scattering microscopy. Nat Biomed Eng 2017;1:0027.

82. Ji M, Lewis S, Camelo-Piragua S, et al. Detection of human brain tumor infiltration with quantitative stimulated Raman scattering microscopy. Sci Transl Med 2015; 7(309). 309ra163.

83. Orillac C, Stummer W, Orringer DA. Fluorescence Guidance and intraoperative Adjuvants to Maximize extent of resection. Neurosurgery 2021;89(5):727–36.

84. Golub D, Hyde J, Dogra S, et al. Intraoperative MRI versus 5-ALA in high-grade glioma resection: a network meta-analysis. J Neurosurg 2020;134(2):484–98.

85. Eyüpoglu IY, Hore N, Savaskan NE, et al. Improving the extent of malignant glioma resection by dual intraoperative visualization approach. PLoS One 2012; 7(9):e44885.

Advances in Imaging to Aid Segmentectomy for Lung Cancer

Kate Krause, MD, Lana Y. Schumacher, MD,
Uma M. Sachdeva, MD, PhD*

KEYWORDS

- Pulmonary segmentectomy • Intraoperative localization • Pulmonary nodules
- Image guidance • Indocyanine green • Near-infrared imaging

KEY POINTS

- Expanded lung cancer screening guidelines have led to enhanced detection of small (<2 cm) pulmonary nodules, prompting the development of adjunct imaging modalities to aid the intraoperative localization of small nodules.
- Pulmonary segmentectomy is gaining acceptance for resection of early-stage lung cancers but is a technically challenging operation which requires surgeons to understand complex segmental and subsegmental anatomy and the potential for vascular anomalies.
- There are multiple options for marking small pulmonary nodules, each with unique advantages, disadvantages, and potential complications.
- Indocyanine green is a safe, inexpensive dye that can be used to demarcate the intersegmental plane, sentinel lymph nodes, and for localization of small pulmonary nodules.
- Three-dimensional computed tomography provides individualized anatomic mapping for preoperative planning and intraoperative navigation.

INTRODUCTION

With the expansion of lung cancer screening criteria, more small pulmonary nodules and early-stage lung cancers are being detected in the United States.[1,2] Although lung cancer remains the leading cause of cancer-related mortality in America, the prognosis is improving,[2-5] and the surgical resection of small, early-stage lesions has become prevalent, with curative intent. In 1995, published results of LCSG821, a randomized trial comparing lobectomy and sublobar resection, including wedge resection or segmentectomy, established lobectomy as the historical surgical standard-of-care treatment for all resectable lung cancers due to improved overall

Division of Thoracic Surgery, Massachusetts General Hospital, 55 Fruit Street, Austen 7, Boston, MA 02114, USA
* Corresponding author.
E-mail address: uma.sachdeva@mgh.harvard.edu

Surg Oncol Clin N Am 31 (2022) 595–608
https://doi.org/10.1016/j.soc.2022.06.003
1055-3207/22/© 2022 Elsevier Inc. All rights reserved.

surgonc.theclinics.com

survival.[6] However, over the past decade, the use of pulmonary segmentectomy for resection of early-stage cancers gained traction, particularly in patients with decreased pulmonary function, advanced age, or comorbidities where the risk associated with lobectomy may be prohibitively high.[7] More recently, the results of JCOG0802, a large prospective randomized clinical trial in Japan comparing the outcomes of segmentectomy and lobectomy for small, early-stage lung cancers, showed that overall survival of patients undergoing segmentectomy was in fact improved relative to those who underwent lobectomy, with nearly identical perioperative morbidity and mortality.[8]

Although debate regarding lobectomy versus segmentectomy remains ongoing, there is a firm trend toward considering segmentectomy as a definitive and standard approach to early-stage lung cancers. The American College of Chest Physicians recently updated their guidelines to state that sublobar resection with negative margins is preferred over lobectomy for patients with clinical stage I, predominantly ground-glass opacity lesions, ≤2 cm in diameter (class 2C recommendation). In addition, sublobar resection is recommended over nonsurgical therapy for patients with clinical stage I non-small cell lung cancer who may tolerate operative intervention but not lobar resection due to decreased pulmonary function or comorbid disease (class 1B).[9]

Pulmonary segmentectomy is a procedure in which one or more contiguous segments of the lung containing the target lesion are removed. It is not only a technically challenging operation but is also conceptually nuanced given the need to carefully plan the oncologic margins, considering the venous and lymphatic drainage of the tumor as well as anatomic variations for any given patient. Pulmonary segments are grossly indistinguishable from their surrounding segments and surgeons use a variety of methods to establish the intersegmental planes. Minimally invasive techniques, including video-assisted thoracoscopic surgery (VATS) and robotic-assisted thoracoscopic surgery (RATS), have been clearly demonstrated to improve postoperative pain control, length of stay, and non-cancer-related mortality, but they pose additional technical challenges due to the inability to palpate lesions of interest with more than a fingertip or the tip of an instrument, underscoring the importance of preoperative mapping of the target tumor's location and the relevant segmental anatomy.[10–12] Historically, demarcation of the intersegmental plane was performed by identifying the inflation–deflation line after occlusion of the target segmental bronchus before division. This technique requires the operative lung to be reinflated following occlusion of the segmental bronchus, enabling the collapsed segmental area to be resected and the inflated parenchyma to be preserved. However, the reproducibility of this maneuver is debated as collateral circulation through the pores of Khon can obscure the inflation–deflation line, which can in turn diminish requisite oncologic margins. This technique can also be difficult when the working space is limited, as may occur with minimally invasive approaches, and can be challenging with emphysematous lungs that require prolonged deflation time of bullous lung tissue.

In parallel with the increased use of segmentectomy in early-stage lung cancers, several techniques relying on advanced imaging and localization strategies have been developed to better identify small, non-palpable tumors and to delineate accurate intersegmental borders. This article reviews the advances in imaging techniques to aid in segmentectomy for lung cancer, focusing on preoperative localization strategies using markers and three-dimensional computed tomography (3D-CT), intraoperative definition of sentinel lymph nodes and the intersegmental plane, and emerging techniques using virtual reality in the robotic platform.

DISCUSSION
Preoperative Planning for Segmentectomy

Although there is minimal variability with regard to pulmonary lobar anatomy, segmental anatomy is highly anomalous and must be well understood by thoracic surgeons in anticipation of sub-lobar resections.[13] When performing pulmonary segmentectomy, identification of the intersegmental plane is of critical importance not only for adequate oncologic margins but also for reducing perioperative complications.[14,15] Each patient's anatomy must be carefully studied from preoperative CT imaging to understand the specific branching pattern of the vessels and bronchi in relation to the target tumor. This has led surgeons to use a variety of imaging and localization techniques to visualize target nodules and relevant pulmonary anatomy at multiple stages throughout the preoperative and intraoperative periods.

Localization Techniques to Mark Small Pulmonary Nodules

There are currently multiple accepted techniques for localization of deep or non-palpable pulmonary nodules. It is common for radiopaque markers to be placed preoperatively through CT-guided and bronchoscopic approaches. In CT-guided percutaneous approaches, interventionalists place fiducials, hookwires, or microcoils into the target lesion, which are then localized intraoperatively using fluoroscopy to identify the site for resection. Local anesthesia and sedation are often needed to improve patient comfort and ensure accurate placement. **Table 1** summarizes the most common percutaneous methods for marking lung nodules, along with their associated advantages, disadvantages, and potential complications.

Solid markers
Fiducials are radiopaque, inert gold markers, usually 3 mm in size, that can be placed percutaneously under CT guidance at, or very near, the lesion of interest. They are then visualized intraoperatively under fluoroscopic guidance to facilitate accurate resection of the target tumor.[16–18] Similarly, microcoils are platinum coils which can be placed preoperatively through a percutaneous, CT-guided approach. Intraoperative identification also requires fluoroscopy (**Fig. 1**), as the microcoils cannot be seen easily with thoracoscopy alone.[19] In addition to percutaneous CT-guided approaches, microcoils can be placed bronchoscopically, which is advantageous when the lesion of interest is near the hilum, or in apical or basal areas that are difficult to safely access percutaneously.[20] Advantages of these techniques include the ability to place markers up to 48 hours before planned surgery, allowing more flexibility in scheduling in settings where operative time is more restricted. Although these placement procedures are generally very well tolerated, patients should be counseled about radiation exposure given the need for intraoperative fluoroscopy. Complication rates are low but include marker migration, pneumothorax, hemothorax, or embolization.[17,18] Confirmation of resection of the target lesion containing the fiducial can be performed immediately in the operating room using specimen radiography (**Fig. 2**).

The hookwire technique is the oldest, and still the most common, marking technique. Placement of a double-barbed wire occurs under direct CT guidance, with the external entry point of the wire chosen as the shortest safe distance to the lesion of interest.[21,22] Once advanced, the tip of the wire is expanded to advance into, or directly adjacent to, the nodule. After confirmation of wire placement with CT, the patient is transferred immediately to the operating room for pulmonary resection. Unlike microcoils and fiducials, fluoroscopy is not needed with hookwires, sparing the associated radiation exposure. The most common complication is migration or dislodgment of the wire, but other reported complications include pneumothorax,

Table 1
Comparison of localization techniques for small pulmonary nodules

Localization Techniques	Advantages	Disadvantages	Complications
Fiducials/microcoils	Simultaneous localization of multiple lesions Flexibility with time of placement and surgery Well-tolerated	Radiation exposure	Pneumothorax Hemorrhage Migration Embolization
Hookwire	Commonly used, widely available	Dislodgment Patient discomfort with wire outside body Immediate surgery required post-placement	Pneumothorax Subcutaneous emphysema Hemorrhage Migration Air embolism
Dye marking (methylene blue, ICG)	Easy to perform Cost-effective No foreign body	Parenchymal diffusion Immediate surgery needed	Anaphylaxis (very rare)
Dye marking (barium)	Easy to perform No foreign body	Radiation exposure	Parenchymal inflammation and pneumonia (at high doses)

hemothorax, air embolism, and pulmonary hemorrhage.[22–24] Multiple case series have shown that intraparenchymal hemorrhage is frequently mild and pneumothorax is often asymptomatic. Given the risk of dislodgement, hookwire placement must occur immediately before surgery and cannot be performed several days in advance.

Although many of these marking techniques allow for temporal separation of marker placement and surgical resection, the advent of hybrid operating rooms offers the promising alternative of integrating procedures for tumor localization and surgical resection. Intraoperative CT-guided lesion localization and resection can be completed in series in one room under a single anesthetic.[25] This combined strategy may decrease the risk for complications such as marker migration and pneumothorax due to decreased patient mobilization and can decrease the time from nodule identification to definitive treatment. Using hybrid operating rooms, nodules can be biopsied as well as marked, enabling diagnosis, localization, and resection within the same setting. This hybrid strategy, however, requires specialized equipment in a dedicated integrated operating suite, which is not currently available at most centers.

Radiofrequency identification tags

Radiofrequency identification (RFID) tags are a developing area of interest for tumor localization. Currently approved for clinical use in Japan, small RFID tags are deployed through the working channel of a bronchoscope, and using navigational bronchoscopy technology, they are placed into a subsegmental bronchus that is adjacent to the tumor.[26–28] The relationship of the tag and tumor is confirmed with CT scan. Marker placement may occur up to 48 hours preoperatively, and more than one marker can be placed, as each tag has a unique identifier. Intraoperatively, the RFID marker is localized using a sterile, handheld probe, and its location can be

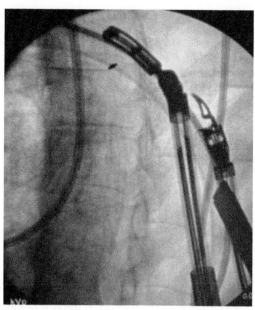

Fig. 1. Fluoroscopic view of microcoil placed before robotic segmentectomy.

monitored in real time as the margins of resection are considered. Some potential concerns with this technology are potential dislodgment of the RFID tag and the need for advanced bronchoscopic skill and access to virtual navigation technology required for placement.

Liquid markers
Methylene blue is a dye which can be injected percutaneously around the margins of a lung nodule under CT guidance, in a procedure similar to placement of microcoils and

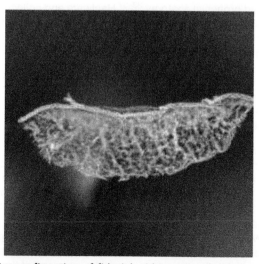

Fig. 2. Intraoperative confirmation of fiducial within resected pulmonary segmentectomy specimen.

fiducial markers; however, no foreign body is left in the lung parenchyma.[29,30] The main challenge is diffusion of the dye into surrounding lung tissue. It is therefore recommended that surgery begin within 120 minutes of dye injection to facilitate accurate localization of the nodule. Methylene blue is a safe, inexpensive dye, though there have been very rare reports of anaphylaxis. It is important to note that the methylene blue dye does not affect histopathologic analysis, however the dye can be difficult to visualize in the setting of anthracotic pigmentation of lung parenchyma.

Barium has also been used to mark lung lesions using CT-guided bronchoscopy and can be performed days before planned surgery given minimal parenchymal diffusion.[31,32] The procedure is technically more difficult but avoids the risks of pneumothorax and hemorrhage associated with percutaneous approaches. There are reports of barium causing acute inflammatory reactions, leading to bronchopneumonia and granuloma formation, both of which could affect the histopathology of the lesion.

Indocyanine green (ICG), a fluorescent dye that will be discussed in more detail below, can also be used to localize small pulmonary nodules through electromagnetic navigation bronchoscopy-guided transbronchial injection, followed by thoracoscopic visualization and resection (**Fig. 3**). Several trials are currently ongoing comparing ICG as a localization strategy to percutaneous hookwire and other techniques using the SPiN Thoracic Navigation System (Veran Medical Technologies). This system combines percutaneous and transbronchial navigation using a Chiba needle with stylet that is inserted percutaneously transthoracically and contains a sensor used for electromagnetic navigation by the bronchoscopic system. This technology can also be used for injection of methylene blue dye or insertion of microcoils.

Three-Dimensional Preoperative and Intraoperative Imaging

Three-dimensional CT bronchography and angiography and virtual-assisted lung mapping (VAL-MAP) using bronchoscopy are preoperative tools that may facilitate the planning of segmental pulmonary resections. Multidetector CT technology has improved access and quality of 3D CT imaging. There are multiple reports describing the use of preoperative and intraoperative models in thoracic surgery to delineate pulmonary vascular and bronchial anatomy.[33–37] Hagiwara and colleagues assessed 124 patients undergoing 3D-CT before pulmonary segmentectomy and found that pulmonary artery (PA) branches were accurately identified in 97.8% of cases, which included 15 cases of anomalous PA branches and 5 cases of anomalous pulmonary vein branches. They also found that patients with 3D imaging had statistically significant improvements in operative time and postoperative complications.[38] The 3D imaging may also be a valuable tool to enhance the learning curve for early career thoracic surgeons and trainees performing pulmonary segmentectomy by enabling improved visualization of pulmonary anatomy and segmental variations.

Virtual-assisted lung mapping

Virtual-assisted lung mapping is a preoperative, bronchoscopic procedure which facilitates lung marking with dye based on virtual images acquired from bronchoscopy. The steps include (1) virtual bronchoscopy with identification of the target bronchus; (2) bronchoscopic lung marking with indigo carmine under direct fluoroscopic guidance; (3) post-marking pulmonary CT with 3D reconstruction; and (4) thoracoscopic lung resection.[39] Most commonly, 2-3 markings are made for wedge resections and 3-4 markings for segmentectomies, which not only allows for better identification of the target lesion but also helps the surgeon map the geometry of the lung parenchyma and plan the resection margins. These markings can be visualized in areas where

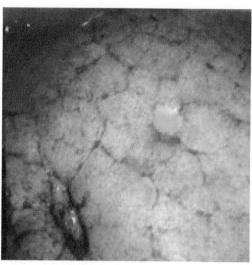

Fig. 3. Intraoperative localization of pulmonary nodule after ICG marking using Veran system.

traditional percutaneous marking approaches are unable to access, including the lung apex, diaphragm, or interlobar fissures. Unlike percutaneous hookwire or coil placement, VAL-MAP does not pose a risk for air embolism, which can be fatal. Sato and colleagues reported their series of 100 consecutive patients undergoing sublobar resection following VAL-MAP, including wedge resection and segmentectomy, and found their technique to be safe, with only four asymptomatic, small pneumothoraces, which is significantly lower than the risk for pneumothorax with hookwires or coils.[40] Sato and colleagues were able to successfully remove 98% of the lesions. They also found that preoperative lung markings were easily identifiable on CT scan 75% of the time, and 98% of the lesions visible on preoperative CT were also visible intraoperatively. Although approximately 25% of markings were not visible, the presence of multiple markings on a given lung meant that surgeons were still able to estimate the target lung segment from the remaining marks, providing an advantage over single marking strategies.

Intraoperative Imaging to Define the Intersegmental Plane and Sentinel Lymph Nodes

ICG is a fluorescent dye used widely across surgical specialties to identify sentinel lymph nodes, define anatomic borders, visualize vascular and lymphatic channels, and evaluate perfusion in surgical anastomoses and tissue flaps. Japanese surgeons pioneered its use in thoracic surgery to identify the intersegmental plane as an alternative to the inflation–deflation technique, which can be unreliable, time-consuming, and particularly challenging when intrathoracic working space is limited.[41,42] ICG is an anionic, nonradioactive, fluorescent dye which binds to plasma proteins. It is excreted by the liver with a half-life of 150-180 seconds and is safe to use in patients with renal failure. Feasibility studies have shown that ICG is safe in humans in systemic doses up to 5 mg/kg, and it is approved by the US Food and Drug Administration for angiography studies and identification of sentinel lymph nodes in multiple cancers. Adverse events are very rare, with the frequency of mild, moderate, and severe side effects 0.15%, 0.2%, and 0.05%, respectively. Anaphylaxis is the most severe complication, and the dye should not be given to patients with known allergy to iodine.[43,44]

To identify the intersegmental plane, ICG is infused intravenously after the surgeon has identified and ligated the target segmental bronchus, artery, and vein. Following injection, the surgical field is visualized with near-infrared fluorescent imaging, which requires use of a fluorescence imaging camera. The isolated pulmonary segment will not receive any dye, whereas the remaining perfused lung will fluoresce when visualized in the near-infrared spectrum (800 nm). The line of demarcation between the dark lung and the fluorescent lung is the intersegmental plane of resection (**Fig. 4**). ICG fluorescence lasts approximately 3-5 minutes.

Yoksukura and colleagues reported their experience using ICG in a cohort of 209 patients at the National Cancer Center in Tokyo and found adequate demarcation of the intersegmental plane in 88% of cases.[45] Successful anatomic delineation was not dependent on the specific resected segment or the absence of obstructive lung disease, and there were no ICG-related adverse events observed. It should be noted that in this study, however, surgeons were free to use high-flow jet ventilation and the inflation–deflation technique if they believed it to be beneficial in determining or confirming the intersegmental plane. If used, the distance between the intersegmental plane identified with jet ventilation and the plane identified with ICG was measured, and they found that the median distance between the planes was 13 mm larger with high-flow jet ventilation compared with ICG. This is likely attributable to collateralization through the pores of Kohn that influence the observed segmental expansion under the inflation–deflation technique. The average time to maximal ICG visualization was 40 seconds, and average time to ICG disappearance was 90 seconds, which highlights the importance of quickly identifying and marking the intersegmental plane with cautery during the period of maximal fluorescence. Surgeons from the Nanjing Chest Hospital also reported a retrospective series of 198 patients undergoing uniportal VATS resections and showed that ICG accurately identified the intersegmental plane in 98% of patients without any increased risk of intraoperative or perioperative complications.[46] They report that the ICG method led to significantly shorter time to identification of the intersegmental planes and decreased overall operative times. Although ICG is most commonly administered intravenously, alternative techniques using transbronchial ICG injection have been reported to be accurate and safe.[47,48] ICG is injected into the peripheral bronchus of the target pulmonary segment and that target segment fluoresces under near-infrared visualization, whereas the remaining lung remains dark.

Overall, utilization of ICG to define the intersegmental plane in pulmonary segmentectomy is increasing, as the dye is safe, nontoxic, readily available, and inexpensive. In retrospective case series, it has been shown to accurately predict the intersegmental plane in 85% to 100% of cases, but larger prospective studies are needed for further evaluation and to reduce selection bias.[41,47,49,50] Misaki and colleagues also report that the technique works well in emphysematous lungs, where the inflation–deflation technique is particularly prone to error.[41] One challenge in the widespread adoption of ICG is that visualization requires the use of an infrared fluorescent imaging system, which may not be universally available. In addition, the plane identified by ICG is often nonlinear and cannot always be easily approximated by a straight staple line.

The use of ICG for identification of sentinel lymph nodes is an emerging area of interest in lung cancer. ICG can be injected transbronchially into the peritumoral region and then identified visually within nodal tissue with near-infrared imaging. Several small studies have shown its safety and feasibility as a marker for lymphatic drainage

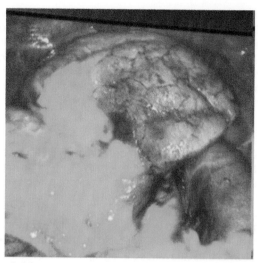

Fig. 4. Delineation of the intersegmental plane using ICG during robotic segmentectomy, with dark (not green) region indicating the target segment for resection.

networks.[51,52] Recently, Digesu and colleagues evaluated the long-term outcomes of sentinel lymph node sampling following peritumoral ICG injection, comparing patients who underwent mediastinal lymph node sampling with and without sentinel lymph node mapping. Not only did they find that sentinel lymph node sampling was 100% specific for local lymph node status, but they report that patients who demonstrated pathologic node-negative disease following sentinel lymph node sampling showed improved disease-free survival as compared with those found to have pathologic node-negative disease by mediastinal lymph node sampling alone. This finding suggests that sentinel lymph node identification and sampling may be more sensitive than non-targeted mediastinal lymph node sampling for identifying true node-positive patients.[53]

Special Considerations for Robotic-Assisted Segmentectomy

RATS is becoming an important part of general thoracic surgery practices. Pulmonary segmentectomy poses anatomic and technical challenges that may be uniquely suited to robotic approaches through the opportunity to integrate preoperative and intraoperative imaging to better delineate patient anatomy. Baste and colleagues describe integration of a 3D imaging platform longitudinally, including preoperative planning, intraoperative navigation, and adjunct procedures including radial endobronchial ultrasound and pleural dye marking.[54] In this paradigm, 3D imaging models are constructed preoperatively and subsequently transmitted to the robotic console intraoperatively and viewed directly beside the live image. The surgeon can then explore and manipulate the 3D model from the robot console to review patient anatomy and immediately adapt the operative plan. Ultimately, the goal is to provide surgeons real-time information to improve surgical decision-making, minimize intraoperative errors, decrease postoperative complications, and improve the surgeon's experience. This has been described by other groups as well, using a variety of imaging software technologies; the main challenges at this juncture are managing the expense, time, and complex workflows involved in the creation and integration of these models across a variety of platforms and into the operating room.[55,56]

Augmented reality lies on the next frontier of imaging technology and robotic surgery, wherein a 3D model of the pulmonary arteries, veins, and bronchi will be integrated within the robotic, intrathoracic view within the console. This technique has been described in hepatic surgery in a few specialized centers.[57] However, this technique will likely prove more challenging to adapt to thoracic surgery, as the deflated operative lung anatomy is not an exact match to the inflated lung map derived from preoperative planning CT images.

SUMMARY

As thoracic surgery continues to advance more minimally invasive techniques, there is an increasing need to optimize visual feedback to the surgeon to improve tumor localization and to better delineate patient anatomy. Pulmonary segmentectomy can be a challenging operation for thoracic surgeons, but it is becoming a standard and arguably favored operation for early-stage lung cancers given the compelling data supporting its oncologic adequacy and decreased morbidity and mortality as compared with lobectomy for early-stage disease. Thoracic surgeons and patients will therefore benefit from integration of these advanced imaging modalities to improve both preoperative planning and intraoperative navigation to localize small nodules, define segmental anatomy, identify the intersegmental plane, and identify draining sentinel lymph node stations.

CLINICS CARE POINTS

- Pulmonary segmentectomy has been associated with improved survival with no increase in morbidity for early-stage non-small cell lung cancers.
- Localization techniques for non-palpable nodules include solid markers (fiducials, microcoils, and hookwires), liquid markers (methylene blue, indocyanine green [ICG], and barium), and radiofrequency identification tags.
- Three-dimensional computed tomography and virtual-assisted mapping have been shown to accurately predict pulmonary vascular branching and segmental anatomic variations.
- ICG is the most widely accepted method for accurate identification of the intersegmental plane during segmental pulmonary resection.

DISCLOSURE

The authors have nothing to disclose.

REFERENCES

1. De Koning H, Van Der Aalst C, Ten Haaf K, et al. Effects of volume CT lung cancer screening: mortality results of the NELSON randomised-controlled population-based trial. J Thorac Oncol 2018;13:S185.
2. National Lung Screening Trial Research Team., Aberle DR, Adams AM, Berg CD, et al. Reduced lung-cancer mortality with low-dose computed tomographic screening. N Engl J Med 2011;365(5):395–409.
3. Siegel R, Naishadham D, Jemal A. Cancer statistics, 2012. CA Cancer J Clin 2012;62:10–29.
4. Cancer Institute National. Cancer Stat Facts: Common Cancer Sites. 2018. Available online: https://seer.cancer.gov/statfacts/html//common.html.

5. Siegel RL, Miller KD, Jemal A. Cancer statistics, 2020. CA Cancer J Clin 2020; 70:7–30.
6. Ginsberg RJ, Rubinstein LV. Randomized trial of lobectomy versus limited resection for T1 N0 non-small cell lung cancer. Lung Cancer Study Group. Ann Thorac Surg 1995;60(3):615–22 ; discussion 622-3.
7. Shirvani SM, Jiang J, Chang JY, et al. Comparative effectiveness of 5 treatment strategies for early-stage non-small cell lung cancer in the elderly. Int J Radiat Oncol Biol Phys 2012;84(5):1060–70.
8. Suzuki K, Saji H, Aokage K, et al. Comparison of pulmonary segmentectomy and lobectomy: Safety results of a randomized trial. J Thorac Cardiovasc Surg 2019; 158:895–907.
9. Howington JA, Blum MG, Chang AC, et al. Treatment of stage I and II non-small cell lung cancer: Diagnosis and management of lung cancer, 3rd ed: American College of Chest Physicians evidence-based clinical practice guidelines. Chest 2013;143:e278S–313S.
10. Bendixen M, Jørgensen OD, Kronborg C, et al. Postoperative pain and quality of life after lobectomy via video-assisted thoracoscopic surgery or anterolateral thoracotomy for early stage lung cancer: a randomised controlled trial. Lancet Oncol 2016;17(6):836–44.
11. Hristov B, Eguchi T, Bains S, et al. Minimally Invasive Lobectomy Is Associated With Lower Noncancer-specific Mortality in Elderly Patients: A Propensity Score Matched Competing Risks Analysis. Ann Surg 2019;270(6):1161–9.
12. Okada M, Mimura T, Ikegaki J, et al. A novel video-assisted anatomic segmentectomy technique: selective segmental inflation via bronchofiberoptic jet followed by cautery cutting. J Thorac Cardiovasc Surg 2007;133(3):753–8.
13. Ohtaki Y, Shimizu K. Anatomical thoracoscopic segmentectomy for lung cancer. Gen Thorac Cardiovasc Surg 2014;62:586–93.
14. Nakamura T, Koide M, Nakamura H, et al. The common trunk of the left pulmonary vein injured incidentally during lung cancer surgery. Ann Thorac Surg 2009;87: 954–5.
15. Akiba T, Marushima H, Kamiya N, et al. Thoracoscopic lobectomy for treated cancer in a patient with an unusual vein anomaly. Ann Thorac Cardiovasc Surg 2011; 17:501–3.
16. Velasquez R, Martin A, Hishmeh MA, et al. Placement of markers or assist minimally invasive resection of peripheral lung lesions. Ann Transl Med 2019; 7(15):350.
17. Sharma A, McDermott S, Mathiesen D, et al. Preoperative localization of lung nodules with fiducial markers: feasibility and technical considerations. Ann Thorac Surg 2017;103(4):1114–20.
18. Sancheti MS, Lee R, Ahmed SU, et al. Percutaneous fiducial localization for thoracoscopic wedge resection of small pulmonary nodules. Ann Thorac Surg 2014; 97:1914–8.
19. Mayo JR, Clifton JC, Powell TI, et al. Lung nodules: CT-guided placement of microcoils to direct video-assisted thoracoscopic surgical resection. Radiology 2009;250(2):576–85.
20. Miyoshi T, Kondo K, Takizawa H, et al. Fluoroscopy-assisted thoracoscopic resection of pulmonary nodules after computed tomography-Guided bronchoscopic metallic coil marking. J Thorac Cardiovasc Surg 2006;131:704–10.
21. Klinkenberg TJ, Dinjens L, Wolf RFE, et al. CT-guided percutaneous hookwire localization increases the efficacy and safety of VATS for pulmonary nodules. J Surg Oncol 2017;115:898–904.

22. Ichinose J, Kohno T, Fujimori S, et al. Efficacy and complications of computed tomography-guided hook wire localization. Ann Thorac Surg 2013;96:1203–8.
23. Kamiyoshihara M, Sakata K, Ishikawa S, et al. Cerebral arterial air embolism following CT-guided lung needle marking. Report of a case. J Cardiovasc Surg (Torino) 2001;42:699–700.
24. Sakiyama S, Kondo K, Matsuoka H, et al. Fatal air embolism during computed tomography-guided pulmonary marking with a hook-type marker. J Thorac Cardiovasc Surg 2003;126:1207–9.
25. Fang H, Chang K, Chao Y. Hybrid operating room for the intraoperative CT-guided localization of pulmonary nodules. Ann Transl Med 2019;7(2):34.
26. Sato T, Yutaka Y, Nakamura T, et al. First clinical application of radiofrequency identification marking system – precise localization of a small lung nodule. Thorac Lung Cancer Evolving Technology 2020;4:301–3.
27. Yutaka Y, Sato T, Zhang J, et al. Localizing small lung lesions in video-assisted thoracoscopic surgery via radiofrequency identification marking. Surg Endosc 2017;31:3353–62.
28. Eguchu T, Sato T, Shimizu K. Technical advances in segmentectomy for lung cancer: A minimally invasive strategy deep, small, and impalpable tumors. Cancers (Basel) 2001;13(13):3137.
29. Lenglinger FX, Schwarz CD, Artmann W. Localization of pulmonary nodules before thoracoscopic surgery: value of percutaneous staining with methylene blue. AJR Am J Roentgenol 1994;163:297–300.
30. Vandoni RE, Cuttat JF, Wicky S, et al. CT-guided methylene-blue labelling before thoracoscopic resection of pulmonary nodules. Eur J Cardiothorac Surg 1998;14:265–70.
31. Kobayashi T, Kaneko M, Kondo H, et al. CT-guided bronchoscopic barium marking for resection of a fluoroscopically invisible peripheral pulmonary lesion. Jpn J Clin Oncol 1997;27:204–5.
32. Okumura T, Kondo H, Suzuki K, et al. Fluoroscopy- assisted thoracoscopic surgery after computed tomography-guided bronchoscopic barium marking. Ann Thorac Surg 2001;71:439–42.
33. Ikeda N, Yoshimura A, Hagiwara M, et al. Three-dimensional computed tomography lung modeling us useful in simulation and navigation of lung surgery. Ann Thorac Cardiovasc Surg 2013;19:1–5.
34. Fukuhara K, Akashi A, Nakane, et al. Preoperative assessment of the pulmonary artery by three-dimensional computed tomograpgy before video-assisted thoracic surgery lobectomy. Eur J Cardiothorac Surg 2008;34:875–7.
35. Saji H, Inoue T, Kato Y, et al. Virtual Segmentectomy based on high-quality three-dimensional computed tomography in a patient with lung cancer undergoing thoracic lobectomy. Gen Thorac Cardiovasc Surg 2008;56:413–6.
36. Watanabe S, Arai K, Watanabe T, et al. Use of three-dimensional computed tomographic angiography of pulmonary vessels for lung resections. Ann Thorac Surg 2003;75:388–92.
37. Nagashima T, Shimizu K, Ohtaki Y, et al. An analysis of variations in the bronchovascular pattern of the right upper lobe using three-dimensional CT angiography and bronchography. Gen Thorac Cardiovasc Surg 2015;63(6):354–60.
38. Hagiwara M, Shimada Y, Kato Y, et al. High-quality 3-dimensional image simulation for pulmonary lobectomy and segmentectomy: results of preoperative assessment of pulmonary vessels and short-term surgical outcomes in consecutive patients undergoing video-assisted thoracic surgery. Eur J Cardio-Thoracic Surg 2014;46(6):e120–6.

39. Sato M, Omasa M, Chen F, et al. Use of virtual assisted lung mapping (VAL-MAP), a bronchoscopic multispot dye-marking technique using virtual images, for precise navigation of thoracoscopic sublobar lung resection. J Thorac Cardiovasc Surg 2014;147:1813–9.

40. Sato M, Yamada T, Menju T, et al. Virtual-assisted lung mapping: outcome of 100 consecutive cases in a single institute. Eur J Cardiothorac Surg 2015;47(4): e131–9.

41. Misaki N, Chang SS, Igai H, et al. New clinically applicable method for visualizing adjacent lung segments using an infrared thoracoscopy system. J Thorac Cardiovasc Surg 2010;140:752–6.

42. Andolfi M, Potenza R, Seguin-Givelet AD. Gossot. Identification of the intersegmental plane during thoracoscopic segmentectomy: state of the art. Interact Cardiovasc Thorac Surg 2020;30(3):329–36.

43. Okusanya OT, Hess NR, Luketich JD, et al. Infrared intraoperative fluorescence imaging using indocyanine green in thoracic surgery. Eur J Cardiothorac Surg 2018;53(3):512–8.

44. Hope-Ross M, Yannuzzi LA, Gragoudas ES. Adverse reactions due to indocyanine green. Ophthalmology 1994;101:529–33.

45. Yotsukura M, Okubbo Y, Yoshida Y, et al. Indocyanine green imaging for pulmonary segmentectomy. JTCVS Tech 2021;6:151–8.

46. Sun Y, Zhang Q, Shao F, et al. Feasibility Investigation of Fluorescence Method in Uniport Thorascopic Anatomical Segmentectomy for Identifying the Intersegmental Boundary Line. Chin J Lung Cancer 2021;24(11):756–63.

47. Sekine Y, Ko E, Oishi H, et al. A simple and effective technique for identification of intersegmental planes by infrared thoracoscopy after transbronchial injection of indocyanine green. J Thorac Cardiovasc Surg 2012;143(6):1330–5.

48. Oh S, Suzuki K, Miyasaka Y, et al. New technique for lung segmentectomy using indocyanine green injection. Ann Thorac Surg 2013;95(6):2188–90.

49. Kasai Y, Tarumi S, Chang SS, et al. Clinical trial of new methods for identifying lung intersegmental borders using infrared thorascopy with indocyanine green: comparative analysis of 2- and 10 wavelength methods. Eur J Cardiothorac Surg 2013;44(6):1103–7.

50. Lizuka S, Kuroda H, Yoshimura K, et al. Predictors of indocyanine green visualization during fluorescence imaging of segmental plane formation in thorascopic anatomical. segmentectomy 2016;8(5):985–91.

51. Yamashita S, Tokuishi K, Anami K, et al. Video-assisted thoracoscopic indocyanine green fluorescence imaging system shows sentinel lymph nodes in non-small-cell lung cancer. J Thorac Cardiovasc Surg 2011;141:141–4.

52. Gilmore DM, Khullar OV, Jaklitsch MT, et al. Identification of metastatic nodal disease in a phase 1 dose-escalation trial of intraoperative sentinel lymph node mapping in non-small cell lung cancer using near-infrared imaging. J Thorac Cardiovasc Surg 2013;146:562–70 ; discussion: 9–70.

53. Digesu CS, Hachey KJ, Gilmore DM, et al. Long-term outcomes after near-infrared sentinel lymph node mapping in non-small cell lung cancer. J Thorac Cardiovasc Surg 2018;155:1280–91.

54. Baste JM, Soldea V, Lachkar S, et al. Development of a precision multimodal surgical navigation system for lung robotic segmentectomy. J Thorac Dis 2018; 10(10).

55. Volonté F, Pugin F, Bucher P, et al. Augmented reality and image overlay navigation with OsiriX in laparoscopic and robotic surgery: not only a matter of fashion. J Hepatobiliary Pancreat Sci 2011;18:506–9.

56. Lachkar S, Baste JM, Guisier F, et al. Pleural dye marking using radial endobronchial ultrasound and virtual bronchoscopy before sublobar pulmonary resection for small peripheral nodules. Eur Respir J 2017;50:PA3779.

57. Ntourakis D, Memeo R, Soler L, et al. Augmented Reality Guidance for the Resection of Missing Colorectal Liver Metastases: An Initial Experience. World J Surg 2016;40:419–26.

Indocyanine Green Use During Esophagectomy

Michael H. Gerber, MD, Stephanie G. Worrell, MD*

KEYWORDS

- Esophagectomy • Perfusion • Imaging • Anastomoses • Gastric conduit

KEY POINTS

- The use of indocyanine green fluorescent angiography (ICG-FA) during esophagectomy is a feasible and safe method to determine conduit perfusion.
- The imaging systems used for FA are available for both minimally invasive surgery and open approaches and display fluorescence in real time.
- Most methods of ICG-FA rely on subjective assessment by surgeons but have rapid and simple interpretation to make intraoperative adjustments that may decrease anastomotic leaks.

INTRODUCTION

Modern esophageal surgery has its beginnings in the nineteenth century but the first transthoracic esophagectomy was performed by Franz Torek in 1913 with the use of an external artificial conduit.[1] The use of a gastric conduit was not popularized until decades later when Ivor Lewis published his 2-staged approach in 1946, McKeown published his 3-hole approach in 1976, and Orringer described his transhiatal resection in 1978.[2–4] One of the major complications of any of these techniques, and usually the most worrisome, is an anastomotic leak, which represents a poor prognostic factor for patients' overall survival.

The 30-day mortality for patients undergoing esophagectomy in the most recent Society of Thoracic Surgeons (STS) general thoracic surgery database analysis was 3.3%.[5] The factors with the highest impact on operative mortality were respiratory distress syndrome, reintubation, renal failure, and anastomotic leak requiring reoperation. Although the leak rate in that study was 12.8%, a separate STS database study looked at leak rates based on the site of the anastomosis and found a cervical anastomosis had a 12.3% anastomotic leak rate versus a 9.3% leak rate with a thoracic anastomosis with both having similar 30-day mortalities, 3.6% and 2.7%,

Department of Surgery, Section of Thoracic Surgery, University of Arizona, 1501 N Campbell Avenue Room #4302, Tucson, AZ 85724, USA
* Corresponding author.
E-mail address: sworrell@arizona.edu

Surg Oncol Clin N Am 31 (2022) 609–629
https://doi.org/10.1016/j.soc.2022.06.008
1055-3207/22/© 2022 Elsevier Inc. All rights reserved.

respectively.[6] Because an anastomotic leak was associated with mortality rates as high as 25% in the 1980s, retrospective studies tried to identify factors associated with anastomotic leak and found albumin lesser than 3g/dL, positive resection margin, and cervical anastomosis were associated with leaks.[7] Anastomotic leaks are not just associated with an increase in 30-day mortality, 7.2% from 3.1% but they are also associated with an increase in morbidity including arrhythmias, deep venous thrombosis, pneumonia, acute respiratory distress syndrome, ventilatory support, empyema, sepsis, stricture, and renal failure.[6] The factors associated with anastomotic leak on multivariate analysis were congestive heart failure, hypertension, renal insufficiency, and cervical anastomosis.

During an esophagectomy, many factors can influence the anastomosis. Surgical factors include anastomotic tension, location of the anastomosis, surgical technique (ie, stapled vs hand sewn, minimally invasive vs open), and perfusion of the conduit. Traditionally when performing gastrointestinal anastomoses, surgeons have relied on subjective findings in the conduit such as determining color of the tissue, evaluating bleeding on the cut edges of the tissue, palpating pulses or obtaining Doppler signals, and assessing peristalsis of the conduit to determine the conduit's perfusion and viability. However, these subjective measures could be misinterpreted, unreliable, and have surgeon variation. One clinical trial assessed surgeon prediction accuracy for anastomotic leak in colorectal anastomoses and found surgeon sensitivity was 38% to 62% and specificity was 46% to 52% depending on the site of anastomosis.[8]

During the past several decades, surgeons have trialed various methods to assess conduit perfusion during esophagectomies. One recent review of objective measurements summarized the available techniques which include: pulse oximetry, polarographic measurement of oxygen tension, near infrared and visible light spectrophotometry, intravital microscopy, Doppler ultrasound, hydrogen gas clearance, radioisotope studies, fluorescence studies, infrared imaging, laser Doppler flowmetry, bowel wall contractility measurements, pH measurement, microdialysis, and assessment of electrical properties.[9] However, only a few of these techniques are feasible, affordable, and trialed in human studies.

The use of indocyanine green (ICG) with fluorescent imaging technology to assess intestinal perfusion has become much more feasible during the past decade due to the available technology, ease of use, and safety.[10–12] This article will discuss the various methods of fluorescent angiography (FA) to determine intestinal perfusion using ICG and fluorescent imaging.

How to Use Indocyanine Green

ICG is a water-soluble, near-infrared fluorophore that has been used in various surgical fields because it provides high sensitivity and good contrast between tissues because it has low inherent autofluorescence background with high tissue penetration. When used for FA, the molecule binds rapidly to plasma proteins in the blood and is quickly cleared by the liver and then excreted in the biliary system. In the bloodstream, the half-life is 2 to 4 minutes and the ICG is usually cleared from blood in 15 to 20 minutes. The ICG excitation spectrum after intravenous (IV) injection ranges from just more than 700 nm to nearly 850 nm. The emission spectrum in blood has a peak range in the 810 to 830 nm.[13] For ICG-FA to become a useful tool in assessing the intestinal conduit's perfusion during esophagectomies, the detection site, detection time, and fluorescent parameters need to be easy to identify, quick to measure, and simple to use.

ICG is readily available and approved for use on human subjects for determining cardiac output, hepatic function and liver blood flow, and for ophthalmic angiography.

The compound is soluble in water, and the lyophilized powder form is easily reconstituted in distilled water and can be further diluted with a saline solution before injection (**Fig. 1**). When used for FA, ICG is typically injected as an IV bolus through either a peripheral IV (pIV) line or central venous line (CVL) followed by a flush to ensure the intended dye is pushed in to the circulation as a bolus. The fluorophore quickly binds to proteins in blood and therefore is typically detectable within seconds. The exact time to fluorescence after injection can be variable and depends on dose, injection site, cardiac output, and hematocrit.[13]

The imaging systems used for FA are available for both minimally invasive surgery and open approaches and display fluorescence in real time. Some equipment has built in software to determine fluorescent intensity (FI) at specific regions of interest. See **Table 1** Imaging Systems for a list of some imaging systems and software used for ICG-FA in esophageal reconstruction.

The dosing of ICG for FA is variable. The total maximum dose for human subjects should be less than 2 mg/kg. Most studies assessing bowel perfusion use a bolus

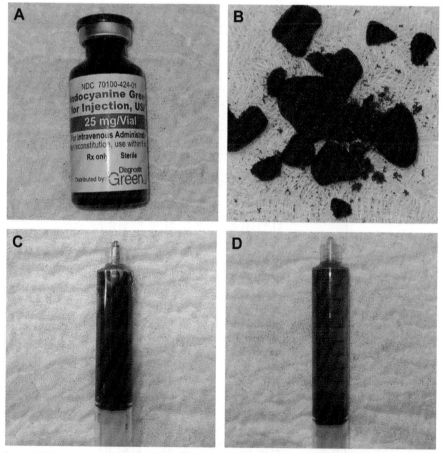

Fig. 1. ICG in a commercial container (*A*), as a lyophilized powder (*B*), reconstituted in water at a concentration of 2.5 mg/mL (*C*), and reconstituted in water at a more dilute concentration of 0.25 mg/mL (*D*).

Table 1
Imaging systems

System	Manufacturer	Available for MIS	Real Time Images	Imaging Overlay	Analysis Software
PhotoDynamic Eye (PDE)	Hamamatsu Photonics K.K. (Hamamatsu, Japan)	No	Yes	No	ROI
HyperEye Medical System (HEMS)	Mizuho Medical Co., Ltd. (Tokyo, Japan)	No	Yes	Yes	LumiView
IC-View	Pulsion Medical Systems (Munich, Germany)	No	Yes	No	IC-Calc
SPY/SPY Elite	Stryker (Kalamazoo, Michigan, USA)	No	Yes	Yes	SPY Q
FireFly	Intuitive Surgical (Sunnyvale, California, USA)	Yes	Yes	No	Not specified
Image1	KARL STORZ (El Segundo, California, USA)	Yes	Yes	Yes	Not specified
PinPoint	Stryker (Kalamazoo, Michigan, USA)	Yes	Yes	Yes	SPY Q
LIGHT VISION	Shimadzu Corp. (Kyoto, Japan)	No	Yes	Yes	Not specified
Fluobeam 800	Fluoptics (Grenoble, France)	No	Yes	No	FluoSoft
VISERA ELITE II	Olympus (Center Valley, Pennsylvania, USA)	Yes	Yes	Yes	Not specified
Oupumandi Fluorescent Endoscope	OptoMedic Technology Co. (Foshan, China)	Yes	Yes	Yes	Not specified

dose between 1.25 and 15 mg although a few studies used weight-based dosing between 0.05 and 0.3 mg/kg as seen in **Table 2**. The dye may be injected multiple times throughout an operation because the bloodstream half-life is short and is cleared from the circulation by the liver typically within 20 minutes (**Fig. 2**A).

Fluorescent angiography during esophagectomy

There are a variety of ways in which surgeons use intraoperative FA to determine perfusion of an intestinal conduit during an esophagectomy. Most studies use FA to assess the gastric conduit once the gastric tube has been created. With open techniques, the gastric tube is usually laid on the anterior chest wall, stretched out toward the head, as if it were laying in its future neo-esophagus orientation allowing the surgeon to determine any perfusion deficits once the ICG is injected. The surgeon is then able to make modifications to the conduit based on perfusion assessment. With minimally invasive techniques, the gastric conduit is either assessed in situ during the abdominal portion of the operation, or later when it is pulled into the thoracic cavity before the anastomosis as described by various studies seen in **Table 2**. Some groups have used other timing of FA. For example, one study injected ICG after the gastric vessels had been ligated but before the gastric tube creation.[14] This timing of FA allows the surgeon to modify the creation of the gastric tube based on perfusion assessment of the gastric conduit. Another study used ICG-FA during the anastomosis to determine sites of suture placement in the anterior portion of the anastomosis.[15] As ICG has a short half-life and is quickly cleared from the circulation, it is possible to use it multiple times throughout the operation if the surgeon wishes to assess the tissue in multiple situations or after modifications have been made.[16,17]

Once the surgeon has used ICG-FA to determine perfusion characteristics, different modifications can be performed in order to reduce leak rates as seen in **Table 3**. The most common conduit modification was to resect the malperfused proximal/cephalad portion of the conduit.[15,17–23] Other groups simply moved the anastomotic site to areas that were considered adequately perfused tissue,[24–27] whereas others adjusted the type of anastomosis they performed, whether it was end-to-end, end-to-side, stapled, or hand sewn.[15,28,29] Another modification strategy was to add additional vascular anastomoses such as an arterial anastomosis to "super-charge" the conduit or add an additional venous anastomosis to increase venous drainage of the conduit.[25,29,30] In practice, surgeons use ICG-FA in many different ways to assess perfusion allowing for specific adjustments to the tissue or surgical technique.

Tissue perfusion assessment techniques

To assess tissue perfusion using ICG-FA, groups have used various subjective and objective methods due to the lack of clear normal values. Subjective measures include visualization of FI and time to adequate fluorescence of the tissues. Objective measurements include flow pattern in the vessels that perfuse the proximal/cephalad conduit,[31–34] flow velocity,[35,36] inflow/outflow patterns using software measurements of FI versus time curves,[16,37,38] and FI with software calculated specific cutoff values for good versus poor perfusion.[24] Many of these objective values are obtained in an effort to set standard numbers for which surgeons may follow for prediction of anastomotic healing. However, using these objective measurements require calculations or the use of software, which may burden the surgeon.

Initial reports using ICG-FA in esophageal surgery tended to use subjective, qualitative measurements of perfusion. Either the tissue had adequate fluorescence to the eye of the surgeon, or it did not. This assessment is akin to prior techniques of perfusion assessment looking at bowel color, bleeding at the tip of the conduit, or

Table 2
Current studies with ICG use during esophagectomy

Reference	Country	Study Design	Enrollment Dates	ICG Dose	ICG Admin Route	Timing of ICG Admin	Imaging System/Distance
Campbell et al,[24] 2015	United States	Retrospective cohort Case control study	2007–2013	5 mg	IV	After conduit creation	SPY Elite (not specified)
Dalton et al,[18] 2018	United States	Retrospective cohort Case control study	2014–2016	7.5 mg	IV	After conduit creation	PINPOINT (not specified)
Hodari et al,[15] 2015	United States	Retrospective cohort Case control study	2011–2014	Not specified	Not specified	After conduit creation	FireFly (not specified)
Ishige et al,[16] 2019	Japan	Prospective cohort Feasibility study	2015–2017	1.25 mg	IV	Predissection; After conduit creation; after pull up	Olympus (1 cm)
Ishiguro et al,[39] 2012	Japan	Case report	Not specified	2.5 mg	pIV	After conduit creation	PDE (not specified)
Ishikawa et al,[38] 2021	United States	Retrospective cohort Case control study	2015–2020	5 mg	IV	After conduit creation	SPY Elite (not specified)
Karampinis et al,[19] 2017	Germany	Retrospective cohort Case control study	2010–2016	7.5 mg	CVL	After conduit creation	PINPOINT (not specified)
Kitagawa et al,[45] 2018	Japan	Retrospective cohort Case control study	2011–2017	5 mg	CVL	Before and after conduit creation	HEMS (not specified)
Kitagawa et al,[17] 2020	Japan	Retrospective cohort Case control study	2016–2020	5 mg	Not specified	Before and after conduit creation	LIGHT VISION (not specified)
Koyanagi et al,[35] 2016	Japan	Prospective cohort Case control study	2014–2015	1.25–2.5 mg	CVL	After conduit creation	PDE (not specified)
Kubota et al,[34] 2013	Japan	Prospective cohort Feasibility study	2010–2011	0.5 g/kg	not specified	After conduit creation	HEMS (50–70 cm)
Kumagai et al,[33] 2014	Japan	Prospective cohort Feasibility study	Not specified	2.5 mg	pIV	After conduit creation	PDE (not specified)
Kumagai[46]	Japan	Prospective cohort Feasibility study	2014–2017	2.5 mg	pIV	After conduit creation	PDE (not specified)

Study	Country	Study design	Years	ICG dose	Route	Timing	Imaging system
Lin et al,[47] 2020	China	Prospective cohort Feasibility study	2018–2020	0.75 mg	pIV	After conduit creation	Oupumandi fluorescent endoscope (20 cm)
Luo et al,[41] 2020	China	Prospective cohort Case control study	2017–2019	0.5 mg/kg (max 25 mg)	CVL	After conduit creation	SPY (20 cm)
Murawa et al,[28] 2012	Poland	Prospective cohort Feasibility study	2009–2010	25 mg	Not specified	After conduit creation	IC-View (not specified)
Noma et al,[25] 2018	Japan	Retrospective cohort Case control study	2010–2016	12.5 mg	CVL	After conduit creation	PDE (not specified)
Ohi et al,[29] 2017, Ohi et al,[32] 2017	Japan	Retrospective cohort Case control study	2000–2015	2.5 mg	Not specified	After conduit creation	PDE (not specified)
Pacheco et al,[40] 2013	United States	Retrospective cohort Feasibility study	2010–2011	Not specified	Not specified	After conduit creation	SPY (not specified)
Pather et al,[20] 2022	United States	Retrospective cohort Feasibility study	2014–2018	7.5 mg	IV	After conduit creation	PINPOINT (not specified)
Rino et al,[31] 2014	Japan	Prospective cohort Feasibility study	2009–2013	2.5 mg	Not specified	After conduit creation	PDE (not specified)
Sarkaria et al,[48] 2014	United States	Prospective cohort Feasibility study	2012–2013	10 mg	pIV	Before conduit creation	FireFly (not specified)
Shimada et al,[30] 2011	United States	Prospective cohort Feasibility study	Not specified	5 mg	Not specified	After conduit creation	IMAGE1 (not specified)
Shimada et al,[30] 2011	Japan	Prospective cohort Feasibility study	2008–2011	2.5 mg	Not specified	After conduit creation	PDE (not specified)
Slooter et al,[26] 2021	The Netherlands	Prospective cohort Feasibility study	2018–2019	0.05 mg/kg	pIV	After conduit creation	PINPOINT/Spy-phi (not specified)
Talavera-Urquijo et al,[36] 2020	Italy	Prospective cohort Feasibility study	2017–2019	0.3 mg/kg	IV	Before and after conduit creation	Olympus (not specified)
Thammineedi et al,[22] 2020	India	Prospective cohort Feasibility study	2019–2019	2.5–15 mg	IV	After conduit creation	PINPOINT (not specified)
Yamaguchi et al,[23] 2021	Japan	Prospective cohort Feasibility study	2017–2019	2.5 mg	IV	After conduit creation	PDE (not specified)

(continued on next page)

Table 2
(continued)

Reference	Country	Study Design	Enrollment Dates	ICG Dose	ICG Admin Route	Timing of ICG Admin	Imaging System/ Distance
Yukaya et al,[37] 2015	Japan	Prospective cohort Feasibility study	2013–2014	0.1 mg/kg	pIV	After conduit creation	HEMS (not specified)
Zehetner et al,[27] 2015	United States	Prospective cohort Case control study	2008–2011	2.5 mg	CVL	After conduit creation	SPY (not specified)

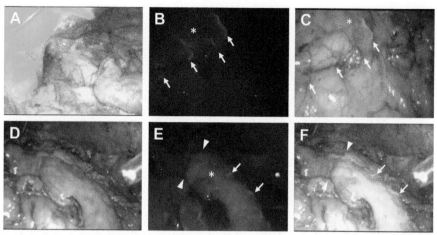

Fig. 2. Laparoscopic images of the gastric conduit using ICG. (*A*) Retained ICG fluorescence seen in the liver 30 minutes after ICG injection with minimal fluorescence in other tissue. (*B-C*) Gastric conduit ICG detection in fluorescent and fused images is first seen in the right gastroepiploic arcade (*arrows*) while tissue microperfusion (*) is not seen as rapidly. (*D-F*) The gastric conduit appears equally well perfused in visible light as seen in (*D*), but ICG-FA (*E-F*) reveals a line of fluorescent demarcation (*arrowheads*) between rapidly perfused conduit and proximal/cephalad delayed perfusion including the both the macroperfusion in the gastroepiploic arcade (*arrows*) and tissue microperfusion (*).

assessing Doppler signals in the conduit. Moreover, one group suggested that there is a learning curve when using ICG-FA to assess perfusion.[27] However, FA does allow the surgeon to see better details of tissue perfusion including which vessels are intact and supplying the proximal/cephalad portion of the conduit, the direction of blood flow in these vessels, and how quickly the tissue (the microvascular network) begins to show fluorescence compared with other regions of the conduit (**Fig. 2**B-F). Several groups mentioned that traditional visual assessment of the conduit missed areas that ICG-FA found to be inadequately perfused.[16,39,40] When comparing Doppler signals to ICG-FA in the conduit, one group noted that the Doppler signal always disappeared distal/caudad to the ICG-FA adequate perfusion line, and Doppler signals were unable to differentiate when the conduit had adequate microperfusion to the proximal/cephalad tip or if there was a malperfused area based on FI demarcation seen with ICG-FA.[27] Thus, even the subjective measurements of ICG-FA to determine tissue perfusion add additional value when assessing intestinal conduit.

The simplest measurement of ICG-FA is to see if the tissue has FI or never develops FI. However, given enough time, most conduits will show some FI even at the most proximal/cephalad portion. Another method is to use specific timepoints and mark the conduit at the border between the fluorescent and nonfluorescent portions of the conduits at those timepoints. This method seems to be the most common and compared with non-ICG assessment decreases the anastomotic leak rate from 10% to 20% to 0% to 8%.[15,24,25,29,41] Using a timepoint is a specific and easy way for the surgeon to quickly assess perfusion of the conduit. However, different centers have different timepoints that show adequate perfusion. Some groups have used a cutoff time after ICG injection as quick as 20 seconds, whereas other groups have used timepoints as long as 120 seconds. Still, some groups categorized perfusion of the conduit based on FI as brisk/ideal after a short timepoint 15 to 60 seconds,

Table 3
ICG-FA use in esophagectomy assessment summary

Reference	Total Patients	Non-ICG Control Patients	Anastomotic Leak/Graft Necrosis	Conduit Type	Anastomotic Site	ICG-FA Assessment	Intervention
Campbell et al,[24] 2015	90	69	ICG: 0 (0%) Control: 12 (17.4%) Total: 12 (13.3%)	Gastric: 90	Thoracic: 90	Timing: 60 s after ICG ROI: 10 cm from pylorus Cutoff: 75% FI at ROI at timepoint	Adjustment of anastomotic site
Dalton et al,[18] 2018	40	20	ICG: 2 (10%) Control: 1 (5%) Total: 3 (10%)	Gastric: 40	Thoracic: 40	Timing: 60 s after ICG ROI: gross FI of conduit Cutoff: lack of visual FI at timepoint	Adjustment of anastomotic site; resection of proximal conduit
Hodari et al,[15] 2015	54	15	ICG: 0 (0%) Control: 3 (20%) Total: 3 (5.6%)	Gastric: 54	Thoracic: 54	Timing: continuous after ICG ROI: gross FI of conduit Cutoff: lack of visual FI	Resection of distal esophagus and proximal conduit; adjust of anterior anastomotic suture line
Ishige et al,[16] 2019	20	0	ICG: 0 (0%) Control: not specified Total: 0 (0%)	Gastric: 20	Cervical: 3 Thoracic: 17	Timing: continuous after ICG ROI: FI vs time curve at anastomotic site Cutoff: not specified	None
Ishiguro et al,[39] 2012	1	0	ICG: 1 (100%) Control: not specified Total: 1 (100%)	Gastric: 1	Cervical: 1	Timing: continuous after ICG ROI: gross FI of conduit Cutoff: lack of visual FI	None
Ishikawa et al,[38] 2021	304	0	ICG: 70 (23.0%) Control: not specified Total: 70 (23.0%)	Gastric: 304	Cervical: 304	Timing: up to 120 s after ICG ROI: FI vs time curve at antrum, tip of conduit and 5 cm proximal Cutoff: not specified	None

Study			Leak rate	Conduit	Anastomosis	Timing/ROI/Cutoff	Action
Karampinis et al,[19] 2017	90	55	ICG: 3 (8.6%) Control: 10 (18.2%) Total: 13 (14.4%)	Gastric: 90	Cervical: 27 Thoracic: 63	Timing: continuous after ICG ROI: gross FI of conduit Cutoff: lack of visual FI	Adjustment of anastomotic site; resection of proximal conduit
Kitagawa et al,[45] 2018	72	0	ICG: 7 (9.7%) Control: not specified Total: 7 (9.7%)	Gastric: 72	Cervical: 72	Timing: continuous after ICG ROI: gross FI of conduit Cutoff: lack of visual FI	Adjustment of anastomotic site; resection of proximal conduit
Kitagawa et al,[17] 2020	66	0	ICG: 10 (15.2%) Control: not specified Total: 10 (15.2%)	Gastric: 66	Cervical: 66	Timing: continuous after ICG, time to FI in abdomen and chest ROI: tip of conduit Cutoff: not specified	None
Koyanagi et al,[35] 2016	40	0	ICG: 7 (17.5%) Control: not specified Total: 7 (17.5%)	Gastric: 40	Cervical: 40	Timing: continuous after ICG, speed of FI ROI: pylorus and tip of conduit Cutoff: not specified	None
Kubota et al,[34] 2013	5	0	ICG: 0 (0%) Control: not specified Total: 0 (0%)	Gastric: 4 Ileo-colonic: 1	Cervical: 5	Timing: continuous after ICG ROI: gross FI of conduit Cutoff: not specified	None
Kumagai et al,[33] 2014	20	0	ICG: 2 (10%) Control: not specified Total: 2 (10%)	Gastric: 20	Cervical: 20	Timing: continuous after ICG ROI: gastroepiploic arcade Cutoff: not specified	None
Kumagai et al,[46] 2018	70	0	ICG: 1 (1.4%) Control: not specified Total: 1 (1.4%)	Gastric: 70	Cervical: 70	Timing: 60 and 90 s after ICG ROI: gross FI of conduit Cutoff: lack of visual FI at timepoints	Adjustment of anastomotic site; resection of proximal conduit

(continued on next page)

Table 3
(continued)

Reference	Total Patients	Non-ICG Control Patients	Anastomotic Leak/Graft Necrosis	Conduit Type	Anastomotic Site	ICG-FA Assessment	Intervention
Lin et al,[47] 2022	84	0	ICG: 8 (9.5%) Control: not specified Total: 8 (9.5%)	Jejunal: 84	Cervical: 16 Thoracic: 68	Timing: continuous after ICG ROI: tip of conduit Cutoff: not specified	None
Luo et al,[41] 202	192	106	ICG: 1 (1.2%) Control: 11 (10.4%) Total: 12 (6.3%)	Gastric: 192	Cervical: 192	Timing: 60 s after ICG ROI: gross FI of conduit Cutoff: lack of visual FI at timepoint	Adjustment of anastomotic site; resection of proximal conduit
Murawa et al,[28] 2012	15	0	ICG: 1 (6.7%) Control: not specified Total: 1 (6.7%)	Gastric: 15	Cervical: 15	Timing: continuous after ICG ROI: gross FI of conduit Cutoff: lack of visual FI	Change to end-to-side anastomosis
Noma et al,[25] 2018	285	214	ICG: 6 (8.5%) Control: 54 (25.2%) Total: 60 (21.1%)	Gastric: 285	Cervical: 285	Timing: 20 and 30 s after ICG ROI: gross FI of conduit Cutoff: lack of visual FI at timepoints	Adjustment of anastomotic site; kocherization performed; addition of arterial/venous anastomoses
Ohi et al,[29] 2017, Ohi et al,[32] 2017	120	61	ICG: 1 (1.7%) Control: 9 (14.8%) Total:10 (8.3%)	Gastric: 120	Cervical: 73 Thoracic: 47	Timing: 15–60 s after ICG ROI: gross FI of conduit Cutoff: lack of visual FI	Change in anastomotic technique; change in surgical approach; addition of arterial/venous anastomoses
Pacheco et al,[40] 2013	11	0	ICG: 2 (18.1%) Control: not specified Total: 2 (18.1%)	Gastric: 11	Cervical: 11	Timing: continuous after ICG ROI: gross FI of conduit Cutoff: not specified	None

Study						
Pather et al,[20] 2022	100	0	ICG: 6 (6%) Control: not specified Total: 6 (6%)	Gastric: 100 Thoracic: 100	Timing: 60 s after ICG ROI: gross Fl of conduit Cutoff: lack of visual Fl at timepoint	Adjustment of anastomotic site; resection of proximal conduit
Rino et al,[31] 2014	33	0	ICG: 5 (15.2%) Control: not specified Total: 5 (15.2%)	Gastric: 33 Thoracic: 33	Timing: continuous after ICG ROI: Left gastroepiploic blood supply Cutoff: not specified	None
Sarkaria et al,[48] 2014	30	0	ICG: 2 (6.7) Control: not specified Total: 2 (6.7%)	Gastric: 30 Cervical: 5 Thoracic: 25	Timing: continuous after ICG ROI: short gastric vasculature Cutoff: not specified	None
Schlottmann[21] 2017	5	0	ICG: 0 (0%) Control: not specified Total: 0 (0%)	Gastric: 5 Thoracic: 5	Timing: continuous after ICG ROI: gross Fl of conduit Cutoff: lack of visual Fl	Adjustment of anastomotic site; resection of proximal conduit
Shimada et al,[30] 2011	40	0	ICG: 3 (7.5%) Control: not specified Total: 3 (7.5%)	Gastric: 36 Jejunal: 3 Ileo-colonic: 1 Cervical: 40	Timing: continuous after ICG ROI: microvasculature of conduit Cutoff: with cutting short gastric vein: improvement in Fl–> additional venous anastomosis; if no Fl improvement–> additional arterial anastomosis	Addition of arterial/venous anastomoses

(continued on next page)

Table 3
(continued)

Reference	Total Patients	Non-ICG Control Patients	Anastomotic Leak/Graft Necrosis	Conduit Type	Anastomotic Site	ICG-FA Assessment	Intervention
Slooter et al,[26] 2021	84	0	ICG: 12 (14.3%) Control: not specified Total: 12 (14.3%)	Gastric: 84	Cervical: 17 Thoracic: 67	Timing: continuous after ICG ROI: gross FI of conduit Cutoff: lack of visual FI	Adjustment of anastomotic site; omental wrapping
Talavera-Urquijo et al,[36] 2020	100	0	ICG: 32 (32%) Control: not specified Total: 32 (32%)	Gastric: 100	Thoracic: 100	Timing: continuous after ICG ROI: gross FI of conduit, base of Right GEA, and stapled edge of conduit Cutoff: not specified	None
Thammineedi et al,[22] 2020	13	0	ICG: 0 (0%) Control: not specified Total: 0 (0%)	Gastric: 13	Cervical: 13	Timing: continuous after ICG ROI: gross FI of conduit and esophagus Cutoff: lack of visual FI	Adjustment of anastomotic site; resection of proximal conduit; additional resection of esophagus
Yamaguchi et al,[23] 2021	129	0	ICG: 4 (3.1%) Control: not specified Total: 4 (3.1%)	Gastric: 129	Cervical: 129	Timing: 60 and 90 s after ICG ROI: gross FI of conduit Cutoff: lack of visual FI at timepoints	Adjustment of anastomotic site; resection of proximal conduit
Yukaya et al,[37] 2015	27	0	ICG: 9 (33.3%) Control: not specified Total: 9 (33.3%)	Gastric: 27	Cervical: 27	Timing: continuous after ICG ROI: last branch of Right GEA and 3 cm proximal Cutoff: not specified	None

						Timing: continuous after ICG ROI: gross FI of conduit Cutoff: lack of visual FI	Adjustment of anastomotic site
Zehetner et al,[27] 2015	144	0	ICG: 24 (16.7%) Control: not specified Total: 24 (16.7%)	Gastric: 144	Cervical: 144		
Summary	2284	540	All ICG: 219 (12.6%) ICG vs control: 13 (3.9%) Control: 100 (18.5%) Total: 319 (14.0%)	Gastric: 2195 (96.1%) Jejunal: 87 (3.8%) Ileo-colonic: 2 (0.1%)	Cervical: 1575 (69.0%) Thoracic: 709 (31.0%)		

moderate/acceptable perfusion after an intermediary timepoint 30 to 90 seconds, and poor/inadequate perfusion after a 60 to 90 second timepoint as seen in **Table 3**. The variations in timepoints for adequate perfusion are likely due to multiple factors: ICG dose, fluorescent imaging equipment, injection through CVL versus pIV, abdominal versus thoracic visualization, length of conduit for cervical versus thoracic anastomosis, and region of interest (ie, tissue microperfusion or vascular arcade perfusion).

Surgeons are trying to find more specific qualitative measurements when using FA to overcome bias when evaluating the conduit. As conduit sizes will vary from person to person, the thought of using a specific universal timepoint across all patients may include some areas of poor perfusion in patients with a short conduit and may exclude areas of good perfusion in patients with a long conduit. To account for this, one study evaluated the speed of fluorescence in gastric conduits.[35] They found the speed of FI in the tissue from the pylorus to the tissue on the lesser curvature at the conduit tip was inversely associated with anastomotic leak. In fact, if the tissue fluorescent speed (tissue microperfusion, not the speed in the gastroepiploic vessels) was more than 1.8 cm/s, there were no anastomotic leaks. Although these measurements put specific numbers on time to fluorescence, the fluorescence is still a subjective measurement, which can vary among individual observers. Surgeons have found ways to combat the subject assessment of fluorescence by using software that can actively measure FI while in the operating room. One group used a single reference point of tissue fluorescence on the gastric conduit 10 cm proximal from the pylorus and measured the FI at this reference point 60 seconds after ICG injection.[24] Areas were considered well perfused if the FI was at least 75% that of the reference point, and all anastomoses were performed in areas of good perfusion. After this technique was implemented, they suffered no anastomotic leaks in the next 21 patients while having 12 (17.4%) of the prior 69 patients leak.

Another method surgeons have implemented to quantitatively characterize tissue perfusion looked at tissue fluorescence curves over time. Specific areas, or regions of interest, on the gastric conduit were picked and using software, the FI over time is measured allowing surgeons to determine flow patterns in the conduit. A group from Michigan performed a post hoc analysis and compared the FI curves at the antrum to the FI curves at the tip of the conduit and an area 5 cm distal/caudad to the conduit tip.[38] They found a significantly lower max FI at the tip and 5 cm distal/caudad to the tip were associated with anastomotic leak, and time to max FI at 5 cm distal to the tip was associated with anastomotic leak. Another group used these FI over time curves to characterize conduit blood flow into 3 categories: normal flow, delayed inflow, and delayed outflow.[37] They found that those with an inflow delay type pattern did not have a visual connection between the left and right gastroepiploic artery but no flow pattern was associated with leak in this small study.

DISCUSSION

This article has discussed much of the published literature on ICG use for FA during esophagectomy. It is important to note, no clinically randomized trial has been performed comparing ICG-FA versus non-ICG to date but Van Daele and colleagues[42] has proposed a single-center study using ICG to evaluate and determine objective measurements that may be used to potentially reduce the incidence of anastomotic leakage. Reviews and meta-analyses have been performed comparing the use of ICG versus non-ICG and found ICG use to have a significantly lower incidence of anastomotic leakage.[11,12,43,44] In fact, 3 recent meta-analyses found the use of ICG during esophagectomy had an overall leak rate of 10% to 11%, and when comparing studies with ICG and non-ICG cohorts, the leak rate is 5% to 6% and 20% to 21%, respectively, with an absolute risk reduction of 70%.[12,43,44] Van Daele and colleagues[12] found 12.4% of patients that underwent ICG-FA had changes in surgical management due to inadequate perfusion with anastomotic leaks occurring in 6.5% of these patients compared with the 6.3% leak rate of patients with adequate ICG perfusion of the anastomosis while those without adequate perfusion on ICG assessment had a 47.8% leak rate. This suggests that ICG-FA can direct intraoperative management of the conduit to place the anastomosis in a well-perfused region to reduce anastomotic leak rates. Similarly, Ladak and colleagues[44] found a leak rate of 5.2% when the anastomosis was in a well-perfused site determined by ICG-FA and 33.6% when the anastomosis was in a poorly perfused site. When evaluating the ICG studies that included a control group, Van Daele and colleagues[12] found that well-perfused anastomoses by ICG-FA had a leak rate of 3.0%, those with changes in surgical plan had a 9.5% leak rate, and those with a poorly perfused anastomotic site had a 100% leak rate, whereas the control group had a 20.5% leak rate. Although these are not randomized studies that are being evaluated in the meta-analyses, the evidence suggests that ICG-FA may reduce the incidence of anastomotic leak or identify patients at high risk of leak to which postoperative management may be tailored to.

Currently, no method of ICG-FA is universally standardized between institutions. Therefore, each institution must develop its own standardized protocol for ICG use during esophagectomy. This begins with the timing of ICG dose, whether to be performed just after vessel ligation and before gastric conduit formation, after gastric tube formation, or at the time of anastomosis. Next, the place where the conduit is assessed needs to be determined, whether the conduit is pulled out onto the chest, is in situ in the abdomen, or is in the neo-esophagus position after pull through into the chest. The imaging system must be consistent, and distance of the conduit to the camera as well as camera angle to the conduit needs to be consistent as these will alter the FI the surgeon observes. Respiratory variation may cause changes in distance from the camera and needs to be accounted for as well. The dose of ICG should be standardized either using weight-based dosing or a single consistent dose among all patients. The route of administration should be consistent as either a pIV bolus or CVL bolus followed by a flush. The institution must be consistent when evaluating the conduit, either the entire conduit is to be grossly visualized or there is to be a specific region(s) of interest where the fluorescence is to be measured. If there is a specific region(s) of interest, it should be standardized considering if the measurement will be on the major blood supply vessels on the greater curvature or on the tissue of the conduit (evaluating the microvasculature) and considering the distance from the pylorus or the distance to the tip of the conduit. If timing is to be measured, T_0 needs to be standardized to the time of ICG injection or first enhancement of the either the gastric conduit or the root of the right gastroepiploic vessel, and so forth. When measuring FI, the surgeons must have a standardized subjective criterion or they may use software measurements giving them objective data. The length of fluorescent recording should be predetermined to be sure all ICG assessments are treated equally. If interventions are planned based on ICG-FA assessment, what are the interventions (change in anastomotic site, change in type of anastomosis, resection of conduit, addition of arterial/venous anastomoses, different postoperative management), and what are the specific criteria for each intervention? There are many different factors to account for when using ICG-FA, and each institution should have a standard protocol allowing for the consistent assessment of FA.

The use of ICG-FA during esophagectomy is a feasible and safe method to determine conduit perfusion. It is quick and simple to use with the appropriate equipment and does not extend the length of the operation. Most methods using ICG-FA are subjective assessments by surgeons but have been shown to have rapid and easy interpretation that is used to make intraoperative adjustments that may decrease anastomotic leaks. Additional software may be used for image processing that gives more quantitative data for surgeon use and can further standardize the ICG-FA assessment of perfusion. ICG has a great potential for use during esophagectomies to help guide surgeon management and reduce patient complications.

DISCLOSURE

The authors have nothing to disclose.

REFERENCES

1. Torek F. The operative treatment of carcinoma of the oesophagus. Ann Surg 1915; 61(4):385–405.
2. Lewis I. The surgical treatment of carcinoma of the oesophagus; with special reference to a new operation for growths of the middle third. Br J Surg 1946; 34:18–31.
3. McKeown KC. Total three-stage oesophagectomy for cancer of the oesophagus. Br J Surg 1976;63(4):259–62.
4. Orringer MB, Sloan H. Esophagectomy without thoracotomy. J Thorac Cardiovasc Surg 1978;76(5):643–54.
5. Linden PA, Towe CW, Watson TJ, et al. Mortality after esophagectomy: analysis of individual complications and their association with mortality. J Gastrointest Surg 2020;24(9):1948–54.
6. Kassis ES, Kosinski AS, Ross P, et al. Predictors of anastomotic leak after esophagectomy: an analysis of the society of thoracic surgeons general thoracic database. Ann Thorac Surg 2013;96(6):1919–26.
7. Patil PK, Patel SG, Mistry RC, et al. Cancer of the esophagus: esophagogastric anastomotic leak–a retrospective study of predisposing factors. J Surg Oncol 1992;49(3):163–7.
8. Karliczek A, Harlaar NJ, Zeebregts CJ, et al. Surgeons lack predictive accuracy for anastomotic leakage in gastrointestinal surgery. Int J Colorectal Dis 2009; 24(5):569–76.
9. Urbanavicius L, Pattyn P, Van de Putte D, et al. How to assess intestinal viability during surgery: a review of techniques. World J Gastrointest Surg 2011;3(5): 59–69.
10. Alander JT, Kaartinen I, Laakso A, et al. A review of indocyanine green fluorescent imaging in surgery. Int J Biomed Imaging 2012;2012:940585.
11. Degett TH, Andersen HS, Gogenur I. Indocyanine green fluorescence angiography for intraoperative assessment of gastrointestinal anastomotic perfusion: a systematic review of clinical trials. Langenbecks Arch Surg 2016;401(6):767–75.
12. Van Daele E, Nieuwenhove YV, Ceelen W, et al. Near-infrared fluorescence guided esophageal reconstructive surgery: a systematic review. World J Gastrointest Oncol 2019;11(3):250–63.
13. Desmettre T, Devoisselle JM, Mordon S. Fluorescence properties and metabolic features of indocyanine green (ICG) as related to angiography. Surv Ophthalmol 2000;45(1):15–27.
14. Kitagawa H, Namikawa T, Munekage M, et al. Visualization of the stomach's arterial networks during esophageal surgery using the hypereye medical system. Anticancer Res 2015;35(11):6201–5.

15. Hodari A, Park KU, Lace B, et al. Robot-assisted minimally invasive ivor lewis esophagectomy with real-time perfusion assessment. Ann Thorac Surg 2015; 100(3):947–52.

16. Ishige F, Nabeya Y, Hoshino I, et al. Quantitative assessment of the blood perfusion of the gastric conduit by indocyanine green imaging. J Surg Res 2019;234: 303–10.

17. Kitagawa H, Namikawa T, Iwabu J, et al. Correlation between indocyanine green visualization time in the gastric tube and postoperative endoscopic assessment of the anastomosis after esophageal surgery. Surg Today 2020;50(11):1375–82.

18. Dalton BGA, Abubaker AA, Crandall M, et al. Near infrared perfusion assessment of gastric conduit during minimally invasive Ivor Lewis esophagectomy. Am J Surg 2018;216(3):524–7.

19. Karampinis I, Ronellenfitsch U, Mertens C, et al. Indocyanine green tissue angiography affects anastomotic leakage after esophagectomy. A retrospective, case-control study. Int J Surg 2017;48:210–4.

20. Pather K, Deladisma AM, Guerrier C, et al. Indocyanine green perfusion assessment of the gastric conduit in minimally invasive Ivor Lewis esophagectomy. Surg Endosc 2022;36(2):896–903.

21. Schlottmann F, Patti MG. Evaluation of gastric conduit perfusion during esophagectomy with indocyanine green fluorescence imaging. J Laparoendosc Adv Surg Tech A 2017;27(12):1305–8.

22. Thammineedi SR, Patnaik SC, Saksena AR, et al. The utility of indocyanine green angiography in the assessment of perfusion of gastric conduit and proximal esophageal stump against visual assessment in patients undergoing esophagectomy: a prospective Study. Indian J Surg Oncol 2020;11(4):684–91.

23. Yamaguchi K, Kumagai Y, Saito K, et al. The evaluation of the gastric tube blood flow by indocyanine green fluorescence angiography during esophagectomy: a multicenter prospective study. Gen Thorac Cardiovasc Surg 2021;69(7):1118–24.

24. Campbell C, Reames MK, Robinson M, et al. Conduit vascular evaluation is associated with reduction in anastomotic leak after esophagectomy. J Gastrointest Surg 2015;19(5):806–12.

25. Noma K, Shirakawa Y, Kanaya N, et al. Visualized evaluation of blood flow to the gastric conduit and complications in esophageal reconstruction. J Am Coll Surg 2018;226(3):241–51.

26. Slooter MD, de Bruin DM, Eshuis WJ, et al. Quantitative fluorescence-guided perfusion assessment of the gastric conduit to predict anastomotic complications after esophagectomy. Dis Esophagus 2021;34(5).

27. Zehetner J, DeMeester SR, Alicuben ET, et al. Intraoperative assessment of perfusion of the gastric graft and correlation with anastomotic leaks after esophagectomy. Ann Surg 2015;262(1):74–8.

28. Murawa D, Hunerbein M, Spychala A, et al. Indocyanine green angiography for evaluation of gastric conduit perfusion during esophagectomy–first experience. Acta Chir Belg 2012;112(4):275–80.

29. Ohi M, Toiyama Y, Mohri Y, et al. Prevalence of anastomotic leak and the impact of indocyanine green fluorescein imaging for evaluating blood flow in the gastric conduit following esophageal cancer surgery. Esophagus 2017;14(4):351–9.

30. Shimada Y, Okumura T, Nagata T, et al. Usefulness of blood supply visualization by indocyanine green fluorescence for reconstruction during esophagectomy. Esophagus 2011;8(4):259–66.

31. Rino Y, Yukawa N, Sato T, et al. Visualization of blood supply route to the reconstructed stomach by indocyanine green fluorescence imaging during esophagectomy. BMC Med Imaging 2014;14:18.

32. Ohi M, Saigusa S, Toiyama Y, et al. Evaluation of blood flow with indocyanine green-guided imaging to determine optimal site for gastric conduit anastomosis to prevent anastomotic leak after esophagectomy. Am Surg 2017;83(6):e197–9.

33. Kumagai Y, Ishiguro T, Haga N, et al. Hemodynamics of the reconstructed gastric tube during esophagectomy: assessment of outcomes with indocyanine green fluorescence. World J Surg 2014;38(1):138–43.

34. Kubota K, Yashida M, Kuroda J, et al. Application of the HyperEye Medical System for esophageal cancer surgery: a preliminary report. Surg Today 2013;43(2):215–20.

35. Koyanagi K, Ozawa S, Oguma J, et al. Blood flow speed of the gastric conduit assessed by indocyanine green fluorescence: New predictive evaluation of anastomotic leakage after esophagectomy. Medicine (Baltimore) 2016;95(30):e4386.

36. Talavera-Urquijo E, Parise P, Palucci M, et al. Perfusion speed of indocyanine green in the stomach before tubulization is an objective and useful parameter to evaluate gastric microcirculation during Ivor-Lewis esophagectomy. Surg Endosc 2020;34(12):5649–59.

37. Yukaya T, Saeki H, Kasagi Y, et al. Indocyanine green fluorescence angiography for quantitative evaluation of gastric tube perfusion in patients undergoing esophagectomy. J Am Coll Surg 2015;221(2):e37–42.

38. Ishikawa Y, Breuler C, Chang AC, et al. Quantitative perfusion assessment of gastric conduit with indocyanine green dye to predict anastomotic leak after esophagectomy. Dis Esophagus 2021.

39. Ishiguro T, Kumagai Y, Ono T, et al. Usefulness of indocyanine green angiography for evaluation of blood supply in a reconstructed gastric tube during esophagectomy. Int Surg 2012;97(4):340–4.

40. Pacheco PE, Hill SM, Henriques SM, et al. The novel use of intraoperative laser-induced fluorescence of indocyanine green tissue angiography for evaluation of the gastric conduit in esophageal reconstructive surgery. Am J Surg 2013;205(3):349–52 [discussion: 352-3].

41. Luo RJ, Zhu ZY, He ZF, et al. Efficacy of indocyanine green fluorescence angiography in preventing anastomotic leakage after mckeown minimally invasive esophagectomy. Front Oncol 2020;10:619822.

42. Van Daele E, Nieuwenhove YV, Ceelen W, et al. Assessment of graft perfusion and oxygenation for improved outcome in esophageal cancer surgery: protocol for a single-center prospective observational study. Medicine (Baltimore) 2018;97(38):e12073.

43. Slooter MD, Eshuis WJ, Cuesta MA, et al. Fluorescent imaging using indocyanine green during esophagectomy to prevent surgical morbidity: a systematic review and meta-analysis. J Thorac Dis 2019;11(Suppl 5):S755–65.

44. Ladak F, Dang JT, Switzer N, et al. Indocyanine green for the prevention of anastomotic leaks following esophagectomy: a meta-analysis. Surg Endosc 2019;33(2):384–94.

45. Kitagawa H, Namikawa T, Iawbu J, et al. Assessment of the blood supply using the indocyanine green fluorescence method and postoperative endoscopic evaluation of anastomosis of the gastric tube during esophagectomy. Surg Endosc 2018;32(4):1749–54.

46. Kumagai Y, Hatano S, Sobajima J, et al. Indocyanine green fluorescence angiography of the reconstructed gastric tube during esophagectomy: efficacy of the 90-second rule. Dis Esophagus 2018;31(12).
47. Lin Z, Sun S, Chen Y, et al. Indocyanine green fluorescence imaging improves the assessment of blood supply of interposition jejunum. Surg Endosc 2022.
48. Sarkaria IS, Bains MS, Finley DJ, et al. Intraoperative near-infrared fluorescence imaging as an adjunct to robotic-assisted minimally invasive esophagectomy. Innovations (Phila) 2014;9(5):391–3.

Innovations in Parathyroid Localization Imaging

Claire E. Graves, MD[a,*], Quan-Yang Duh, MD[b], Insoo Suh, MD[c]

KEYWORDS

- Fluorocholine PET • Parathyroid autofluorescence
- Contrast-enhanced fluorescence

KEY POINTS

- Accurate identification of parathyroid glands is critical during cervical procedures, both to remove abnormal and preserve normal glands.
- A variety of preoperative parathyroid imaging techniques are used for identification of abnormal parathyroid glands. New radiotracers for functional PET imaging, paired with CT or MRI for precise anatomic mapping, are demonstrating superior accuracy compared with traditional modalities.
- Parathyroid glands have autofluorescent properties when excited with near-infrared light. New techniques, including commercially available image-based and probe-based devices, have harnessed this property for intraoperative identification of parathyroid tissue.
- Additional techniques have been described to assess intraoperative parathyroid perfusion, typically using fluorescent contrast agents, to predict postoperative function.
- New technologies continue to expand the field of parathyroid imaging.

INTRODUCTION

Parathyroid hormone (PTH), produced by the parathyroid glands, maintains the body's calcium homeostasis. Typically, 2 parathyroid glands are located posterior or adjacent to each lobe of the thyroid. The upper glands usually lie posterior to the recurrent laryngeal nerve near the tracheoesophageal groove, whereas the lower glands are along the posterolateral border of the inferior thyroid pole. Normal parathyroid glands are approximately the size of a grain of rice, and each gland is enclosed within a connective tissue capsule and surrounded by fat and lymph nodes, which can make identification challenging. In addition, the locations of parathyroid glands can vary. The

[a] Department of Surgery, Section of Endocrine Surgery, University of California Davis, 4501 X Street, Suite 3010, Sacramento, CA 95817, USA; [b] Department of Surgery, Section of Endocrine Surgery and Professor, University of California San Francisco, 1600 Divisadero St., San Francisco, CA 94115, USA; [c] Department of Surgery, NYU Langone Health, 530 First Avenue, Suite 6H, New York, NY 10016, USA
* Corresponding author.
E-mail address: cegraves@ucdavis.edu

Surg Oncol Clin N Am 31 (2022) 631–647
https://doi.org/10.1016/j.soc.2022.06.004

lower glands tend to have more variable anatomy and can be located anterior, inferior, or lateral to the lower pole of the thyroid, within the cervical portion of the thymus, within the anterior mediastinum, or even within the thyroid gland.[1]

Localization and identification of parathyroid glands is necessary during cervical surgery—either to remove hyperfunctioning, abnormal glands in patients with hyperparathyroidism or to preserve normal glands during surgery for other purposes (eg, thyroidectomy). In parathyroid surgery, preoperative imaging can help guide surgeons to abnormal glands targeted for resection. Dedicated parathyroid imaging is not performed before thyroidectomy, and the glands are identified intraoperatively by visual inspection. Needle aspiration for PTH measurement and frozen section biopsy are intraoperative adjuncts for confirmation of parathyroid tissue, but neither method helps surgeons to localize parathyroid glands or ensure an intact blood supply. Moreover, both needle aspiration and frozen section analysis require additional time and cost.[2] The challenging nature of parathyroid localization has fostered innovation in imaging techniques to localize glands both before and during cervical operations.

Preoperative Parathyroid Localization

Parathyroidectomy is the only definitive treatment of primary hyperparathyroidism, a disorder of one or more parathyroid glands resulting in overproduction of PTH. Although localization of an abnormal gland (or glands) is not a requirement before parathyroidectomy, preoperative localization can aid in operative planning and execution, can identify ectopic and/or supernumerary glands, and is essential before consideration of minimally invasive or focused parathyroidectomy.[3,4] In reoperative surgery for persistent or recurrent hyperparathyroidism, preoperative localization is necessary to limit dissection and minimize risks of surgery in a reoperative field.[5]

Cervical ultrasound, performed by an experienced parathyroid sonographer, is widely used as an initial imaging study in primary hyperparathyroidism. It is recommended before cervical exploration by the American Association of Endocrine Surgeons, both to localize abnormal parathyroid glands and to assess for coexisting thyroid disease.[6] However, there is no consensus regarding an optimal algorithm for preoperative parathyroid imaging, and ultimately the type of imaging used is left to the discretion of each clinician based on preference, patient factors, and regional capability and expertise.[6,7] In addition to ultrasound, commonly used imaging modalities include technetium Tc99m sestamibi scintigraphy ("sestamibi"), multiphase computed tomography (CT) neck with and without intravenous contrast ("4D-CT"), and hybrid techniques such as sestamibi single-photon emission computed tomography, usually combined with CT. Multiple imaging modalities may be used in combination to improve accuracy, but for each of these modalities, multigland disease and coexisting thyroid disease can decrease sensitivity.[7]

In the mid-1990s, the use of PET for preoperative localization of abnormal parathyroid glands was first reported, using 2-deoxy-2-[^{18}F]fluoro-D-glucose (FDG)[8] and L-[methyl-^{11}C]-methionine.[9] The use of PET for parathyroid imaging was investigated by only a limited number of centers over the subsequent 20 years, likely due to variable results with FDG PET, the limited availability of ^{11}C-methionine, and high cost.[10,11] However, in 2012, Mapelli and colleagues reported an incidental finding of a parathyroid adenoma in a patient undergoing ^{11}C-choline PET/CT for imaging of metastatic prostate cancer.[12] The next year, a similar incidental finding was reported with the use of ^{18}F-fluorocholine, also performed for prostate cancer imaging.[13] Although the mechanism of parathyroid uptake of choline analogues is not fully understood, choline is a marker for cellular proliferation and a precursor to phosphatidylcholine, a phospholipid component of the cell membrane. The increased uptake in abnormal parathyroid glands is hypothesized to be related to the upregulation of phospholipid/Ca^{2+}-dependent choline kinase in hypercellular parathyroid tissue.[14,15]

Although the use of multiple other tracers has been reported, including [^{11}C]2-hydroxy-N,N,N- trimethylethanaminium, 6-[^{18}F] fluoro-L-DOPA, and N-[(^{18}F)Fluoromethyl]-2-hydroxy-N,N-dimethylethanaminium, ^{11}C-methionine and ^{18}F-fluorocholine have been studied most extensively.[16] Because of its short physical half-life, the use of ^{11}C is restricted to facilities with an on-site cyclotron, and therefore, its use has been more limited compared with ^{18}F-fluorocholine.[14] Moreover, ^{11}C has a higher average positron energy, generating more noise compared with ^{18}F.[14] A comparative meta-analysis of ^{11}C-methionine and ^{18}F-fluorocholine,[17] as well as a small series with direct head-to-head comparison of the 2 modalities,[18] both demonstrated superior sensitivity of ^{18}F-fluorocholine (92% vs 80% pooled sensitivity, $P < .01$), with similar positive predictive values (94% vs 95%, $P = .99$).[17]

Since their incidental discovery, multiple centers have investigated the use of ^{18}F-fluorocholine or ^{11}C-choline PET imaging for patients with hyperparathyroidism.[19–21] A systematic review including 23 publications and 1112 patients demonstrated higher diagnostic accuracy of ^{18}F-fluorocholine PET/CT compared with cervical ultrasound as well as multiple sestamibi protocols.[21] Benefits of choline-analogue PET tracers over Tc99m sestamibi parathyroid scintigraphy include superior spatial resolution, more rapid acquisition, and lower radiation exposure. Although predominantly paired with low-dose CT for anatomic correlation, ^{18}F-fluorocholine PET/MRI has also demonstrated promising diagnostic accuracy with the added benefit of avoiding excess ionizing radiation (**Fig. 1**A).[22–24]

^{18}F-fluorocholine PET/CT and PET/MRI demonstrate particularly promising results among patients with negative, equivocal, or discordant results on standard imaging[22,25–29]; reoperative patients[30,31]; or patients with multiple parathyroid adenomas or hyperplasia.[32,33] Currently, due to lower availability and higher cost, these modalities are primarily used as second-line techniques for patients who fail to localize on first-line imaging. However, the improved sensitivity afforded by ^{18}F-fluorocholine PET has led some providers to advocate for its use as a first-line, "one-stop-shop" for preoperative parathyroid localization.[33,34] Although larger-scale studies and cost-effectiveness analyses will be necessary to support this proposed clinical algorithm, preliminary cost models for the United States demonstrate favorable results for ^{18}F-fluorocholine PET as a cost-effective imaging option.[35]

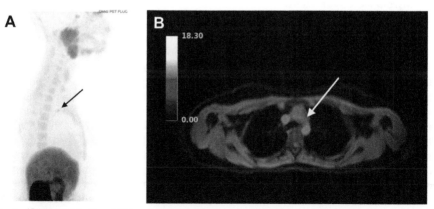

Fig. 1. ^{18}F-fluorocholine PET image of an ectopic mediastinal parathyroid adenoma (*arrows*) on (*A*) sagittal and (*B*) axial view fused with simultaneous MRI.

INTRAOPERATIVE PARATHYROID IDENTIFICATION

Intraoperative identification of parathyroid glands is not only required in dedicated parathyroid surgery but is also important for preservation of gland function in central neck procedures for other indications—most commonly, thyroidectomy. Hypoparathyroidism, a decrease in circulating PTH as a result of impaired parathyroid function, is the most common complication in total thyroidectomy and reoperative thyroid surgery. The median incidence of temporary (lasting 6 months or less) hypoparathyroidism following thyroidectomy is approximately 27%.[36,37] Hypoparathyroidism can be caused by deliberate or inadvertent removal of the parathyroid glands, as well as injury during dissection or disruption of the glands' delicate vasculature. Clinically, hypoparathyroidism leads to hypocalcemia, which causes neuromuscular excitability and cardiac electrical instability due to decreased threshold for muscle and nerve cell depolarization. Early symptoms include numbness or tingling of the digits and perioral region, as well as muscle cramping or spasms. More severe nerve excitation can lead to seizures. Cardiovascular consequences of hypocalcemia include QT prolongation that can result in torsades de pointes. Although transient hypoparathyroidism can be effectively treated with oral calcium, permanent hypoparathyroidism requires lifelong therapy and can lead to significant morbidity and increased mortality.[38,39]

During thyroidectomy, surgeons aim to preserve all 4 parathyroid glands, although resection may sometimes be necessary based on the extent of thyroid disease. Gland preservation depends on accurate identification of parathyroid tissue, which is often challenging even for experienced surgeons. Normal parathyroid glands are very small, approximately 2 to 5 mm in diameter, and similar in color to the surrounding thyroid, lymph nodes, and fatty tissue. Incidental parathyroidectomy has been noted in approximately 16% to 22% of thyroid surgeries.[40–43]

In recent years, multiple technologies have been described to assist surgeons in identifying parathyroid glands in "real-time" during surgery. These technologies include optical fiber-based[44,45] or imaging-based[46–48] techniques to identify parathyroid glands based on their autofluorescent properties, optical coherence tomography,[49] laser speckle contrast imaging,[50] Raman spectroscopy,[51] and injection of visible or fluorescent dyes including methylene blue,[52] 5-aminolevulinic acid,[53] carbon nanoparticles,[54] and contrast-enhanced fluorescence imaging using indocyanine green (ICG).[55]

Parathyroid Autofluorescence

Fluorescence occurs when a substance absorbs radiation (in the form of visible light or radiographs) at a shorter wavelength, then emits it at a longer wavelength. "Fluorophores," chemical compounds with fluorescent properties, naturally occur in some tissues, causing "autofluorescence" when excited by an external light source. Intrinsic near-infrared autofluorescence (NIRAF) of parathyroid glands was first described in 2011 by researchers at Vanderbilt University.[56] They found that parathyroid fluorescence in both normal and hyperfunctioning glands was consistently higher than that of surrounding tissues. The responsible compound, or "fluorophore," for NIRAF within the parathyroid glands remains unknown, but no contrast agent is required. Autofluorescence has been found to persist after parathyroid resection and even after formalin fixation or cryopreservation, indicating that it is a result of a chemical structure inherent to the gland and does not depend on perfusion or viability.[57–59]

Identification and assessment of parathyroid NIRAF can be performed by either probe-based or image-based methods. The probe-based method uses a fiber-optic probe connected to a console containing a near-infrared (NIR) diode laser, detector, and interactive display to collect and analyze autofluorescent signal. Image-based systems use an NIR excitation and collection "camera," which then displays images on a monitor. Currently, there are 2 clinical devices that have received clearance by the US Food and Drug Administration (FDA) and Conformite Eurpëenne marking that use NIRAF for real-time detection of parathyroid tissue: the image-based Fluobeam® (Fluoptics, Grenoble, France) and the probe-based PTeye™ system (Medtronic, Minneapolis, MN, USA).[60,61] In addition, other commercial[62–64] and laboratory-built[65] systems have been described to capture and assess parathyroid autofluorescence.

The image-based Fluobeam system uses an NIR (wavelength of 750 nm) laser via a hand-held device to excite tissue within the operative field and collect wavelengths greater than 800 nm for display as video images on a screen in real time (**Figs. 2**, and **3**).[57] The reported sensitivity of the device ranges from 94% to 100%.[57,58,66] In an international multicenter trial, nearly half (46%) of parathyroid glands were identified with NIRAF first before being identified with the naked eye.[66] A single-center randomized trial of patients undergoing total thyroidectomy found that a higher number of parathyroid glands were detected in the NIRAF group compared with standard care (3.5 vs 2.6, $P < .01$). The incidence of hypocalcemia (serum calcium < 7.5 mg/dL) was significantly lower in the NIRAF group (1.2% vs 11.8%, $P < .01$).[67] In a subsequent multicenter randomized trial of patients undergoing total thyroidectomy, the rate of postoperative hypocalcemia, defined as corrected calcium level less than 8.0 mg/dL during hospitalization, was significantly lower in the NIRAF group (9.1% vs 21.7%, $P = .007$), and NIRAF was associated with reduced risk of hypocalcemia (odds ratio = 0.35) in multivariate analyses adjusting for center and surgeon heterogeneity and confounders.[68] In this study, the number of inadvertently resected parathyroid glands was also significantly lower in the NIRAF group.

Because autofluorescence does not depend on gland viability and persists ex-vivo, image-based NIRAF has also been described for use on resected thyroid specimens to scan for parathyroid tissue not identified during surgical resection (**Fig. 4**). In a study of 116 lobectomy specimens considered free of parathyroid tissue after dissection, 12 glands were discovered on surgeon visual examination and subsequently reimplanted and an additional 13 glands were identified using NIRAF autofluorescence, confirmed by surgeon and pathologic evaluation.[69] Notably, an additional 15 glands were identified only on final pathology, all under thyroid tissue at least 2 mm thick. Overall, of the

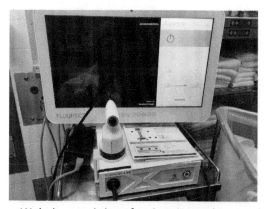

Fig. 2. The Fluobeam LX device, consisting of an imaging probe, console, and touchscreen display.

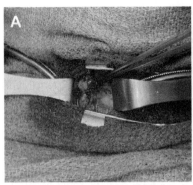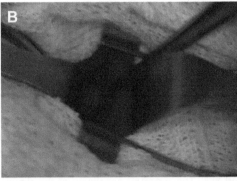

Fig. 3. White light (*A*) and autofluorescence (*B*) images of a normal right upper parathyroid left in situ following right thyroid lobectomy, marked by surgical forceps.

40 unintentionally removed glands, approximately one-third were able to be identified only with the use of autofluorescence and could have been salvaged for autotransplantation.[70]

A meta-analysis of 7 studies comparing the use of NIRAF with Fluobeam with standard treatment found a lower incidence of hypocalcemia at 1 day postoperatively in patients in whom NIRAF was used (relative risk = 0.49, $P < .01$), but there was no significant difference in severe hypocalcemia requiring calcium and vitamin D supplementation or in hypocalcemia 6 months after surgery. Inadvertent parathyroid gland resection was lower in the NIRAF group, with pooled relative risk of 0.48, $P = .02$, but there was no significant association between NIRAF and parathyroid autotransplantation.[71]

The probe-based PTeye system involves a sterile disposable fiber-optic probe joined to a console enclosing an NIR diode laser, detector, and interactive display

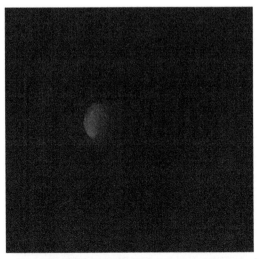

Fig. 4. A subcapsular, normal parathyroid gland is detected with image-based near-infrared autofluorescence ex vivo following total thyroidectomy. This gland was not discovered during dissection with white light, but once identified, it was dissected and autotransplanted.

(Fig. 5). The tip of the probe is touched to the target tissue, and the laser is activated by a foot pedal. The adjoining console then displays a quantitative measurement of fluorescence, as well as the ratio between the tissue and a background baseline (set at the beginning of each case). The system gives an auditory signal if the target tissue's fluorescence is 120% of the background or higher.[2,72] The precommercial system demonstrated a peak parathyroid fluorescence of 1.2 to 29 times thyroid fluorescence, with an overall accuracy of 97%.[73] The reported sensitivities of the probe-based PTeye device, as well as its prototypes and laboratory-built precursors, range from 96% to 100%.[44,72,74,75] An investigation of clinical factors that may affect parathyroid fluorescence found that patient body mass index, preoperative calcium and vitamin D levels, and disease state (malignant vs benign thyroid disease, hyperthyroidism, or hyperparathyroidism) do have an effect on parathyroid fluorescence, whereas patient age, gender, ethnicity, and PTH levels had no effect.[73]

A recent meta-analysis of NIR autofluorescence (pooling data from a variety of both image-based and probe-based systems) as a tool for identification of parathyroid glands during thyroidectomy and parathyroidectomy demonstrated a pooled sensitivity of 0.97, specificity of 0.93, negative predictive value of 0.95, and positive predictive value of 0.95.[76] Subgroup analyses demonstrated similar sensitivity and specificity between probe-based and image-based technology. The probe-based group showed lower positive predictive value (0.92 vs 0.98, $P = .05$) but higher negative predictive value (0.98 vs 0.89, $P = .01$) than the image-based subgroup.

Additional autofluorescence-based techniques have also been described using ultraviolet excitation as opposed to NIR. Multispectral fiber-based fluorescence lifetime imaging (FLIm) uses a handheld laser-induced fluorescence probe to record and measure spectroscopic differences in tissue type. In a pilot study of patients undergoing thyroid and parathyroid surgery, FLIm was able to distinguish parathyroid glands from adjacent thyroid and lymphoid tissue with 100% sensitivity and 93% specificity.[77] Dynamic optical contrast imaging is an image-based technique using light-emitting diodes to acquire images of target tissue in order to detect fluorescence decay and map differences in decay rates.[48] Ex vivo studies demonstrate significant

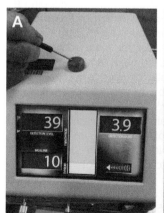
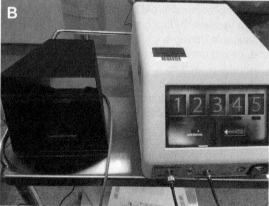

Fig. 5. The PTeye system includes a disposable, sterile, fiber-optic probe, connected to a console containing an NIR diode laser, detector, and interactive display. The tip of the probe touches the tissue to be examined (*A*), and the laser is activated by a foot pedal (*B*), left side of photo.

contrast between parathyroid glands and surrounding tissue,[78] but clinical studies are still pending.

Contrast-Enhanced Parathyroid Fluorescence

Autofluorescence is inherent to the chemical structure of parathyroid gland tissue and therefore unable to evaluate tissue perfusion or viability. However, with the addition of intravascular fluorescent contrast dye or imaging techniques such as laser speckle contrast imaging, NIR light can be used to assess blood flow to the glands. The most frequently described contrast agent is ICG, a fluorescent dye originally developed by Kodak Research Laboratories for use in NIR photography in 1955 and approved for clinical use in 1956.[79] When injected intravenously, ICG binds to plasma proteins, which confines the dye within the vasculature until it is taken up by hepatocytes and excreted into bile. These properties have made ICG clinically useful for angiography, evaluation of tissue perfusion, and hepatobiliary imaging.[80–82] ICG does not target parathyroid tissue specifically, but because the glands are well vascularized and receive more blood flow than the surrounding tissue, the intravascular dye highlights this contrast, demarcating the borders of the gland.[83] Although generally safe and well tolerated, rare adverse reactions have been reported, with an estimated overall incidence of 0.3% to 0.4% and severe reactions occurring in 0.05% to 0.07%.[84,85] The injection solution contains sodium iodide, leading many practitioners to avoid use in patients with iodine allergy.[79]

There are multiple commercially available NIR fluorescence imaging cameras that can be used to acquire images—typically both in grayscale and in combined white light with fluorescence overlay views. These systems do not yet provide real-time quantification of fluorescence, but visual scores have been described to assess gland perfusion. Most commonly, the following system is used: grade 0 = not vascularized (black), grade 1 = moderately vascularized (gray), and grade 2 = well vascularized (white).[86–88] Recently, analyses of dynamic perfusion curves have been suggested, which may more accurately predict gland viability.[89]

During thyroidectomy, ICG fluorescence imaging can be performed both early in the thyroidectomy dissection to identify parathyroid glands and at completion of the dissection to assess perfusion (and therefore viability) of the parathyroid glands left in situ. Contrast-enhanced fluorescence has also been described for mapping the often-complex parathyroid vasculature, in order to guide dissection and preservation of these vessels.[90] During parathyroidectomy, fluorescence imaging can be particularly valuable during subtotal parathyroidectomy. Typically, the most normal-looking gland, based on visual evaluation of its color, size, and shape, is left intact or chosen for subtotal resection. ICG fluorescence imaging can also be used to confirm viability of the remaining parathyroid gland or remnant, thereby theoretically decreasing the risk of permanent postoperative hypoparathyroidism.[91]

Clinical trials suggest ICG-mediated parathyroid evaluation can predict postoperative parathyroid function. A randomized clinical trial of 146 total thyroidectomy patients with at least one well-perfused parathyroid gland with ICG imaging demonstrated noninferiority in the group randomized to no calcium or vitamin D supplementation compared with standard follow-up with postoperative bloodwork and systematic supplementation.[92] No hypocalcemia or hypoparathyroidism was observed in either group at postoperative day 10. Of 50 additional patients in whom no well-perfused parathyroid gland was identified during thyroidectomy, 11 (22%) presented with hypoparathyroidism on postoperative day one, and 6 (12%) on postoperative day 10. One patient had persistent hypoparathyroidism at 6 months after surgery. A similarly designed randomized study of 56 patients demonstrated comparable results, suggesting postoperative calcium, and PTH measurements were not necessary if at least one well-perfused parathyroid gland was observed on ICG evaluation.[93] However, these results are not universal. One study of 86 patients undergoing ICG fluorescence imaging during thyroidectomy found that the sensitivity of at least one well perfused parathyroid gland in predicting normal postoperative PTH was only 58%; 2 or more well-perfused glands increased the sensitivity, but only to 72%.[94]

A meta-analysis of 21 studies with a total of 1309 participants investigating the use of ICG fluorescence for detection of parathyroid glands found an overall sensitivity, specificity, negative predictive value, and positive predictive value of ICG-based detection of parathyroid glands of 93.8%, 83.6%, 73.0%, and 96.7%, respectively.[88] There was no difference in accuracy between manufacturers. When parathyroid ICG fluorescence intensity was scored, there was a significantly lower incidence of hypoparathyroidism on postoperative days 1 and 10 in the high-score group compared with the low-score group.

Recently, laser speckle contrast imaging has been described for assessment of parathyroid vascularity. This label-free imaging technique analyzes superficial blood flow by assessing differences in laser light scatter between adjacent tissues. A recent clinical trial of this technique identified a contrast threshold to assess gland perfusion with an 87.5% sensitivity and 84.4% specificity. Similar to findings from contrast-enhanced fluorescence studies, the study showed that only one vascularized gland determined by laser speckle contrast imaging was needed for normal postoperative PTH.[50]

DISCUSSION

Exciting innovations in preoperative and intraoperative parathyroid localization continue to emerge. Although imaging is not used for the *diagnosis* of primary hyperparathyroidism, preoperative imaging can guide surgeons during exploration, rule out an ectopic gland, and, when appropriate, allow for focused or minimally invasive parathyroidectomy. Traditionally dominant modalities of preoperative parathyroid imaging such as ultrasound and sestamibi, as well as more recent techniques such as 4D-CT, demonstrate regional and institutional variability, and no one strategy has emerged as clearly superior; this may be due, at least in part, to variability in how images are obtained and read at different centers. Practitioner skill and experience has been demonstrated to increase the likelihood of successful localization imaging.[95,96] The optimal modality would allow for easy image acquisition and straightforward interpretation; this is the promise of parathyroid PET, particularly in the settings of negative or discordant results on standard imaging, multiple parathyroid adenomas or hyperplasia, or reoperative patients. Although data collection is ongoing, parathyroid PET imaging has the potential to offer a straightforward protocol and better results in these challenging patient populations, which could allow for more universally accurate imaging.

Real-time intraoperative detection of parathyroid glands using autofluorescence or angiographic techniques is emerging as a useful adjunct for the identification and preservation of parathyroid glands during cervical procedures. Both image-based and probe-based autofluorescence systems have been shown to be accurate, but the 2 techniques each have advantages and disadvantages. The image-based technique displays a field of view that can be useful to identify and map the location of parathyroid glands, even when they have not yet been visually identified by the surgeon under white light. However, the device requires the surgeon to accurately estimate the optimal distance from target tissue for image collection and to visually interpret the resulting images, introducing operator dependence. The probe-based device, in contrast, quantifies fluorescent intensity and provides an audible "yes/no" signal, decreasing user variability. However, as opposed to capturing a wide field of view for parathyroid "mapping," the probe must be precisely placed on target tissue, requiring the surgeon to first identify suspected tissue, then test for confirmation.

A particularly promising application of these intraoperative technologies is for use in surgical education. High-volume cervical surgery and years of experience improve rates of parathyroid identification and preservation during thyroidectomy,[97] but the visual assessment of subtle variations in gross pathology can be challenging to teach trainees. As educational adjuncts for residents or less experienced surgeons in training, parathyroid fluorescence techniques can provide real-time assistance in parathyroid identification as well as, in the case of fluorescence angiography, their feeding vessels.

An important consideration for all the emerging techniques discussed here is the added cost and resources they require. PET imaging is significantly more expensive than ultrasound, sestamibi scintigraphy, SPECT/CT, or 4D-CT. As mentioned earlier, preliminary analysis of expected cost models for the United States suggest that the superior accuracy of ^{18}F-fluorocholine PET may justify the additional cost and make it a cost-effective modality.[35] However, ^{18}F-fluorocholine is not yet approved for commercial use in the United States, and therefore pricing is not yet known. A multicenter randomized trial comparing upfront ^{18}F-fluorocholine PET/CT versus MIBI SPECT/CT has been proposed in France to investigate which modality is the most cost-efficient first-line imaging technique for patients with primary hyperparathyroidism.[98]

Regarding intraoperative localization techniques, current FDA-approved commercial devices require upfront investment for hardware plus per-procedure costs for consumables (sterile sheath for Fluobeam and sterile probe for PTeye). Modifications of readily available equipment[46] and laboratory-built devices[64,99] may also provide lower-cost alternatives. With more than 80,000 total thyroidectomies and parathyroidectomies estimated to be performed in the United States every year—numbers that are expected to increase[100–102]—even a small reduction in surgical complications through accurate and efficient parathyroid identification with fluorescent technologies could have a positive economic impact.[74] Moreover, benefits from the educational aspect of these techniques could be long-term and wide-reaching. Further investigations into the clinical benefits and cost-effectiveness of these techniques are anticipated.

SUMMARY

During cervical surgery, localization and identification of parathyroid glands is key to both the removal of abnormal hyperfunctioning glands and the preservation of normal glands. The challenging nature of parathyroid localization has fostered innovation in imaging techniques to localize glands both before and during cervical operations. Advances in preoperative imaging include PET-based imaging modalities paired with CT or MRI for anatomic correlation. During surgery, parathyroid autofluorescence, contrast-enhanced fluorescence, and fluorescence angiography techniques are useful adjuncts for intraoperative identification.

CLINICS CARE POINTS

- In hyperparathyroidism, preoperative localization can aid in operative planning and execution, can identify ectopic and/or supernumerary glands, and is essential before consideration of minimally invasive or focused parathyroidectomy. It is also necessary for reoperative patients to focus surgical dissection and decrease operative risks.

- ^{18}F-fluorocholine PET/CT and PET/MRI demonstrate promising results for accurate preoperative parathyroid localization, particularly among patients with negative, equivocal, or discordant results on standard imaging, patients with multiple parathyroid adenomas or hyperplasia, and reoperative patients.
- Intraoperative identification of parathyroid glands is critical during thyroidectomy and other cervical procedures to preserve gland function and prevent postoperative hypoparathyroidism.
- The recent discovery of parathyroid gland autofluorescence has led to the development of both image-based and probe-based techniques that can be used as surgical adjuncts during cervical procedures for the identification of parathyroid tissue.
- Techniques to assess parathyroid gland perfusion and viability, including contrast-enhanced fluorescence and laser speckle contrast imaging, can help predict postoperative parathyroid function.

DISCLOSURE

Dr C.E. Graves and Dr Q.Y. Duh have nothing to disclose. Dr I. Suh is a consultant for Prescient Surgical, Medtronic, and Iota Biosciences.

REFERENCES

1. Herrera MF, Gamboa-Dominguez A. Parathyroid Embryology, Anatomy, and Pathology. In: Textbook of Endocrine surgery. 3rd edition. Jaypee Brothers Medical Publishers; 2016. p. 627–36.
2. Solórzano CC, Thomas G, Berber E, et al. Current state of intraoperative use of near infrared fluorescence for parathyroid identification and preservation. Surgery 2021;169(4):868–78.
3. Westerdahl J, Bergenfelz A. Unilateral versus bilateral neck exploration for primary hyperparathyroidism: five-year follow-up of a randomized controlled trial. Ann Surg 2007;246(6):976–80 [discussion; 980-981].
4. Udelsman R, Lin Z, Donovan P. The Superiority of Minimally Invasive Parathyroidectomy Based on 1650 Consecutive Patients With Primary Hyperparathyroidism. Ann Surg 2011;253(3):585–91.
5. Parikh AM, Grogan RH, Morón FE. Localization of Parathyroid Disease in Reoperative Patients with Primary Hyperparathyroidism. Int J Endocrinol 2020; 2020:9649564.
6. Wilhelm SM, Wang TS, Ruan DT, et al. The American Association of Endocrine Surgeons Guidelines for Definitive Management of Primary Hyperparathyroidism. JAMA Surg 2016;151(10):959–68.
7. Zander D, Bunch PM, Policeni B, et al, Expert Panel on Neurological Imaging. ACR Appropriateness Criteria® Parathyroid Adenoma. J Am Coll Radiol 2021; 18(11S):S406–22.
8. Neumann DR, Esselstyn CB, MacIntyre WJ, et al. Parathyroid adenoma localization by PET FDG. J Comput Assist Tomogr 1993;17(6):976–7.
9. Hellman P, Ahlström H, Bergström M, et al. Positron emission tomography with 11C-methionine in hyperparathyroidism. Surgery 1994;116(6):974–81.
10. Beggs AD, Hain SF. Localization of parathyroid adenomas using 11C-methionine positron emission tomography. Nucl Med Commun 2005;26(2):133–6.
11. Weber T, Maier-Funk C, Ohlhauser D, et al. Accurate preoperative localization of parathyroid adenomas with C-11 methionine PET/CT. Ann Surg 2013;257(6): 1124–8.

12. Mapelli P, Busnardo E, Magnani P, et al. Incidental finding of parathyroid adenoma with 11C-choline PET/CT. Clin Nucl Med 2012;37(6):593–5.

13. Quak E, Lheureux S, Reznik Y, et al. F18-choline, a novel PET tracer for parathyroid adenoma? J Clin Endocrinol Metab 2013;98(8):3111–2.

14. Petranović Ovčariček P, Giovanella L, Carrió Gasset I, et al. The EANM practice guidelines for parathyroid imaging. Eur J Nucl Med Mol Imaging 2021;48(9): 2801–22.

15. Ishizuka T, Kajita K, Kamikubo K, et al. Phospholipid/Ca2+-dependent protein kinase activity in human parathyroid adenoma. Endocrinologia japonica 1987; 34(6):965–8.

16. Kluijfhout WP, Pasternak JD, Drake FT, et al. Use of PET tracers for parathyroid localization: a systematic review and meta-analysis. Langenbecks Arch Surg 2016;401(7):925–35.

17. Bioletto F, Barale M, Parasiliti-Caprino M, et al. Comparison of the diagnostic accuracy of 18F-Fluorocholine PET and 11C-Methionine PET for parathyroid localization in primary hyperparathyroidism: a systematic review and meta-analysis. Eur J Endocrinol 2021;185(1):109–20.

18. Mathey C, Keyzer C, Blocklet D, et al. 18F-fluorocholine PET/CT is more sensitive than 11C-methionine PET/CT for the localization of hyperfunctioning parathyroid tissue in primary hyperparathyroidism. J Nucl Med 2021. https://doi.org/10.2967/jnumed.121.262395.

19. Boccalatte LA, Higuera F, Gómez NL, et al. Usefulness of 18F-Fluorocholine Positron Emission Tomography-Computed Tomography in Locating Lesions in Hyperparathyroidism: A Systematic Review. JAMA Otolaryngol Head Neck Surg 2019. https://doi.org/10.1001/jamaoto.2019.0574.

20. Treglia G, Piccardo A, Imperiale A, et al. Diagnostic performance of choline PET for detection of hyperfunctioning parathyroid glands in hyperparathyroidism: a systematic review and meta-analysis. Eur J Nucl Med Mol Imaging 2019; 46(3):751–65.

21. Evangelista L, Ravelli I, Magnani F, et al. 18F-choline PET/CT and PET/MRI in primary and recurrent hyperparathyroidism: a systematic review of the literature. Ann Nucl Med 2020;34(9):601–19.

22. Kluijfhout WP, Pasternak JD, Gosnell JE, et al. 18F Fluorocholine PET/MR Imaging in Patients with Primary Hyperparathyroidism and Inconclusive Conventional Imaging: A Prospective Pilot Study. Radiology 2017;284(2):460–7.

23. Hope TA, Graves CE, Calais J, et al. Accuracy of 18F-fluorocholine PET for the detection of parathyroid adenomas: prospective single center study. J Nucl Med 2021. https://doi.org/10.2967/jnumed.120.256735.

24. Graves CE, Hope TA, Kim J, et al. Superior sensitivity of 18F-fluorocholine: PET localization in primary hyperparathyroidism. Surgery 2022;171(1):47–54.

25. Huber GF, Hüllner M, Schmid C, et al. Benefit of 18F-fluorocholine PET imaging in parathyroid surgery. Eur Radiol 2018;28(6):2700–7.

26. Michaud L, Burgess A, Huchet V, et al. Is 18F-fluorocholine-positron emission tomography/computerized tomography a new imaging tool for detecting hyperfunctioning parathyroid glands in primary or secondary hyperparathyroidism? J Clin Endocrinol Metab 2014;99(12):4531–6.

27. Quak E, Blanchard D, Houdu B, et al. F18-choline PET/CT guided surgery in primary hyperparathyroidism when ultrasound and MIBI SPECT/CT are negative or inconclusive: the APACH1 study. Eur J Nucl Med Mol Imaging 2018;45(4): 658–66.

28. Grimaldi S, Young J, Kamenicky P, et al. Challenging pre-surgical localization of hyperfunctioning parathyroid glands in primary hyperparathyroidism: the added value of 18F-Fluorocholine PET/CT. Eur J Nucl Med Mol Imaging 2018;45(10): 1772–80.

29. Piccardo A, Trimboli P, Rutigliani M, et al. Additional value of integrated 18F-choline PET/4D contrast-enhanced CT in the localization of hyperfunctioning parathyroid glands and correlation with molecular profile. Eur J Nucl Med Mol Imaging 2019;46(3):766–75.

30. Christakis I, Khan S, Sadler GP, et al. 18Fluorocholine PET/CT scanning with arterial phase-enhanced CT is useful for persistent/recurrent primary hyperparathyroidism: first UK case series results. Ann R Coll Surg Engl 2019;101(7): 501–7.

31. Latge A, Riehm S, Vix M, et al. 18F-Fluorocholine PET and 4D-CT in Patients with Persistent and Recurrent Primary Hyperparathyroidism. Diagnostics (Basel) 2021;11(12):2384.

32. Lezaic L, Rep S, Sever MJ, et al. (1)(8)F-Fluorocholine PET/CT for localization of hyperfunctioning parathyroid tissue in primary hyperparathyroidism: a pilot study. Eur J Nucl Med Mol Imaging 2014;41(11):2083–9.

33. Cuderman A, Senica K, Rep S, et al. 18F-Fluorocholine PET/CT in Primary Hyperparathyroidism: Superior Diagnostic Performance to Conventional Scintigraphic Imaging for Localization of Hyperfunctioning Parathyroid Glands. J Nucl Med 2020;61(4):577–83.

34. Giovanella L, Bacigalupo L, Treglia G, et al. Will 18F-fluorocholine PET/CT replace other methods of preoperative parathyroid imaging? Endocrine 2021; 71(2):285–97.

35. Yap A, Hope TA, Graves CE, et al. A cost-utility analysis of 18F-fluorocholine-positron emission tomography imaging for localizing primary hyperparathyroidism in the United States. Surgery 2021;00651–6. https://doi.org/10.1016/j.surg. 2021.03.075. S0039-6060(21).

36. Orloff LA, Wiseman SM, Bernet VJ, et al. American Thyroid Association Statement on Postoperative Hypoparathyroidism: Diagnosis, Prevention, and Management in Adults. Thyroid 2018;28(7):830–41.

37. Edafe O, Antakia R, Laskar N, et al. Systematic review and meta-analysis of predictors of post-thyroidectomy hypocalcaemia. Br J Surg 2014;101(4):307–20.

38. Bergenfelz A, Nordenström E, Almquist M. Morbidity in patients with permanent hypoparathyroidism after total thyroidectomy. Surgery 2020;167(1):124–8.

39. Almquist M, Ivarsson K, Nordenström E, et al. Mortality in patients with permanent hypoparathyroidism after total thyroidectomy. Br J Surg 2018;105(10): 1313–8.

40. Gourgiotis S, Moustafellos P, Dimopoulos N, et al. Inadvertent parathyroidectomy during thyroid surgery: the incidence of a complication of thyroidectomy. Langenbecks Arch Surg 2006;391(6):557–60.

41. Rix TE, Sinha P. Inadvertent parathyroid excision during thyroid surgery. Surgeon 2006;4(6):339–42.

42. Khairy GA, Al-Saif A. Incidental parathyroidectomy during thyroid resection: incidence, risk factors, and outcome. Ann Saudi Med 2011;31(3):274–8.

43. Zhou HY, He JC, McHenry CR. Inadvertent parathyroidectomy: incidence, risk factors, and outcomes. J Surg Res 2016;205(1):70–5.

44. McWade MA, Paras C, White LM, et al. A novel optical approach to intraoperative detection of parathyroid glands. Surgery 2013;154(6):1371–7 [discussion; 1377].

45. Thomas G, McWade MA, Nguyen JQ, et al. Innovative surgical guidance for label-free real-time parathyroid identification. Surgery 2019;165(1):114–23.

46. Ladurner R, Sommerey S, Arabi NA, et al. Intraoperative near-infrared autofluorescence imaging of parathyroid glands. Surg Endosc 2017;31(8):3140–5.

47. Kim SW, Lee HS, Ahn YC, et al. Near-Infrared Autofluorescence Image-Guided Parathyroid Gland Mapping in Thyroidectomy. J Am Coll Surg 2018;226(2):165–72.

48. Kim IA, Taylor ZD, Cheng H, et al. Dynamic Optical Contrast Imaging. Otolaryngol Head Neck Surg 2017;156(3):480–3.

49. Ladurner R, Hallfeldt KKJ, Al Arabi N, et al. Optical coherence tomography as a method to identify parathyroid glands. Lasers Surg Med 2013;45(10):654–9.

50. Mannoh EA, Thomas G, Baregamian N, et al. Assessing Intraoperative Laser Speckle Contrast Imaging of Parathyroid Glands in Relation to Total Thyroidectomy Patient Outcomes. Thyroid 2021. https://doi.org/10.1089/thy.2021.0093. thy.2021.0093.

51. Das K, Stone N, Kendall C, et al. Raman spectroscopy of parathyroid tissue pathology. Lasers Med Sci 2006;21(4):192–7.

52. Dudley NE. Methylene blue for rapid identification of the parathyroids. Br Med J 1971;3(5776):680–1.

53. Prosst RL, Weiss J, Hupp L, et al. Fluorescence-Guided Minimally Invasive Parathyroidectomy: Clinical Experience with a Novel Intraoperative Detection Technique for Parathyroid Glands. World J Surg 2010;34(9):2217–22.

54. Shi C, Tian B, Li S, et al. Enhanced identification and functional protective role of carbon nanoparticles on parathyroid in thyroid cancer surgery: A retrospective Chinese population study. Medicine (Baltimore) 2016;95(46):e5148.

55. Demarchi MS, Karenovics W, Bédat B, et al. Intraoperative Autofluorescence and Indocyanine Green Angiography for the Detection and Preservation of Parathyroid Glands. J Clin Med 2020;9(3). https://doi.org/10.3390/jcm9030830.

56. Paras C, Keller M, White L, et al. Near-infrared autofluorescence for the detection of parathyroid glands. J Biomed Opt 2011;16(6):067012.

57. De Leeuw F, Breuskin I, Abbaci M, et al. Intraoperative Near-infrared Imaging for Parathyroid Gland Identification by Auto-fluorescence: A Feasibility Study. World J Surg 2016;40(9):2131–8.

58. Abbaci M, De Leeuw F, Breuskin I, et al. Parathyroid gland management using optical technologies during thyroidectomy or parathyroidectomy: A systematic review. Oral Oncol 2018;87:186–96.

59. Moore EC, Rudin A, Alameh A, et al. Near-infrared imaging in re-operative parathyroid surgery: first description of autofluorescence from cryopreserved parathyroid glands. Gland Surg 2019;8(3):283–6.

60. Commissioner O of the. FDA permits marketing of two devices that detect parathyroid tissue in real-time during surgery. FDA. 2020. Available at: https://www.fda.gov/news-events/press-announcements/fda-permits-marketing-two-devices-detect-parathyroid-tissue-real-time-during-surgery. Accessed August 5, 2020.

61. Voelker R. Devices Help Surgeons See Parathyroid Tissue. JAMA 2018;320(21):2193.

62. Alesina PF, Meier B, Hinrichs J, et al. Enhanced visualization of parathyroid glands during video-assisted neck surgery. Langenbecks Arch Surg 2018;403(3):395–401.

63. Squires MH, Jarvis R, Shirley LA, et al. Intraoperative Parathyroid Autofluorescence Detection in Patients with Primary Hyperparathyroidism. Ann Surg Oncol 2019;26(4):1142–8.
64. Serra C, Silveira L, Canudo A, et al. Parathyroid identification by autofluorescence – preliminary report on five cases of surgery for primary hyperparathyroidism. BMC Surg 2019;19. https://doi.org/10.1186/s12893-019-0590-9.
65. Kim SW, Song SH, Lee HS, et al. Intraoperative Real-Time Localization of Normal Parathyroid Glands With Autofluorescence Imaging. The J Clin Endocrinol Metab 2016;101(12):4646–52.
66. Kahramangil B, Dip F, Benmiloud F, et al. Detection of Parathyroid Autofluorescence Using Near-Infrared Imaging: A Multicenter Analysis of Concordance Between Different Surgeons. Ann Surg Oncol 2018;25(4):957–62.
67. Dip F, Falco J, Verna S, et al. Randomized Controlled Trial Comparing White Light with Near-Infrared Autofluorescence for Parathyroid Gland Identification During Total Thyroidectomy. J Am Coll Surg 2019;228(5):744–51.
68. Benmiloud F, Godiris-Petit G, Gras R, et al. Association of Autofluorescence-Based Detection of the Parathyroid Glands During Total Thyroidectomy With Postoperative Hypocalcemia Risk: Results of the PARAFLUO Multicenter Randomized Clinical Trial. JAMA Surg 2019. https://doi.org/10.1001/jamasurg.2019.4613.
69. Bellier A, Wazne Y, Chollier T, et al. Spare Parathyroid Glands During Thyroid Surgery with Perioperative Autofluorescence Imaging: A Diagnostic Study. World J Surg 2021;45(9):2785–90.
70. Duh QY, Graves CE. It Helps to Know Where to Look: Visual Identification of Unintentionally Resected Parathyroid Glands is Improved When Inspection is Directed by Near Infrared Autofluorescence Imaging. World J Surg 2021;45(9):2791–2.
71. Wang B, Zhu CR, Liu H, et al. The Ability of Near-Infrared Autofluorescence to Protect Parathyroid Gland Function During Thyroid Surgery: A Meta-Analysis. Front Endocrinol (Lausanne) 2021;12:714691.
72. Thomas G, McWade MA, Paras C, et al. Developing a Clinical Prototype to Guide Surgeons for Intraoperative Label-Free Identification of Parathyroid Glands in Real Time. Thyroid 2018;28(11):1517–31.
73. McWade MA, Sanders ME, Broome JT, et al. Establishing the clinical utility of autofluorescence spectroscopy for parathyroid detection. Surgery 2016;159(1):193–202.
74. Solórzano CC, Thomas G, Baregamian N, et al. Detecting the Near Infrared Autofluorescence of the Human Parathyroid: Hype or Opportunity? Ann Surg 2019. https://doi.org/10.1097/SLA.0000000000003700.
75. Thomas G, Squires MH, Metcalf T, et al. Imaging or Fiber Probe-Based Approach? Assessing Different Methods to Detect Near Infrared Autofluorescence for Intraoperative Parathyroid Identification. J Am Coll Surg 2019;229(6):596–608.e3.
76. Kim DH, Lee S, Jung J, et al. Near-infrared autofluorescence-based parathyroid glands identification in the thyroidectomy or parathyroidectomy: a systematic review and meta-analysis. Langenbecks Arch Surg 2021. https://doi.org/10.1007/s00423-021-02269-8.
77. Marsden M, Weaver SS, Marcu L, et al. Intraoperative Mapping of Parathyroid Glands Using Fluorescence Lifetime Imaging. J Surg Res 2021;265:42–8.
78. Hu Y, Han AY, Huang S, et al. A Tool to Locate Parathyroid Glands Using Dynamic Optical Contrast Imaging. Laryngoscope 2021;131(10):2391–7.

79. Alander JT, Kaartinen I, Laakso A, et al. A review of indocyanine green fluorescent imaging in surgery. Int J Biomed Imaging 2012;2012:940585.

80. Slooter MD, Mansvelders MSE, Bloemen PR, et al. Defining indocyanine green fluorescence to assess anastomotic perfusion during gastrointestinal surgery: systematic review. BJS Open 2021;5(2):zraa074.

81. van den Bos J, Schols RM, Luyer MD, et al. Near-infrared fluorescence cholangiography assisted laparoscopic cholecystectomy versus conventional laparoscopic cholecystectomy (FALCON trial): study protocol for a multicentre randomised controlled trial. BMJ open 2016;6(8):e011668.

82. Majlesara A, Golriz M, Hafezi M, et al. Indocyanine Green Fluorescence Imaging in Hepatobiliary Surgery. Photodiagnosis photodynamic Ther 2016.

83. DeLong JC, Ward EP, Lwin TM, et al. Indocyanine green fluorescence-guided parathyroidectomy for primary hyperparathyroidism. Surgery 2018;163(2):388–92.

84. Obana A, Miki T, Hayashi K, et al. Survey of complications of indocyanine green angiography in Japan. Am J Ophthalmol 1994;118(6):749–53.

85. Hope-Ross M, Yannuzzi LA, Gragoudas ES, et al. Adverse reactions due to indocyanine green. Ophthalmology 1994;101(3):529–33.

86. Vidal Fortuny J, Belfontali V, Sadowski SM, et al. Parathyroid gland angiography with indocyanine green fluorescence to predict parathyroid function after thyroid surgery. Br J Surg 2016;103(5):537–43.

87. Razavi AC, Ibraheem K, Haddad A, et al. Efficacy of indocyanine green fluorescence in predicting parathyroid vascularization during thyroid surgery. Head Neck 2019;41(9):3276–81.

88. Kim DH, Kim SH, Jung J, et al. Indocyanine green fluorescence for parathyroid gland identification and function prediction: Systematic review and meta-analysis. Head Neck 2021. https://doi.org/10.1002/hed.26950.

89. Noltes ME, Metman MJH, Heeman W, et al. A Novel and Generic Workflow of Indocyanine Green Perfusion Assessment Integrating Standardization and Quantification Toward Clinical Implementation. Ann Surg 2021;274(6):e659–63.

90. Benmiloud F, Penaranda G, Chiche L, et al. Intraoperative Mapping Angiograms of the Parathyroid Glands Using Indocyanine Green During Thyroid Surgery: Results of the Fluogreen Study. World J Surg 2022;46(2):416–24.

91. Zaidi N, Bucak E, Okoh A, et al. The utility of indocyanine green near infrared fluorescent imaging in the identification of parathyroid glands during surgery for primary hyperparathyroidism. J Surg Oncol 2016;113(7):771–4.

92. Vidal Fortuny J, Sadowski SM, Belfontali V, et al. Randomized clinical trial of intraoperative parathyroid gland angiography with indocyanine green fluorescence predicting parathyroid function after thyroid surgery. Br J Surg 2018;105(4):350–7.

93. Jin H, Cui M. Research on Intra-Operative Indocyanine Green Angiography of the Parathyroid for Predicting Postoperative Hypoparathyroidism: A Noninferior Randomized Controlled Trial. Endocr Pract 2020;26(12):1469–76.

94. Rudin AV, McKenzie TJ, Thompson GB, et al. Evaluation of Parathyroid Glands with Indocyanine Green Fluorescence Angiography After Thyroidectomy. World J Surg 2019;43(6):1538–43.

95. Yeo CT, Tharmalingam S, Pasieka JL. The value of dynamic surgeon-directed imaging in the preoperative planning of patients with primary hyperparathyroidism. Surgery 2021;169(3):519–23.

96. Zia S, Sippel RS, Chen H. Sestamibi Imaging for Primary Hyperparathyroidism: The Impact of Surgeon Interpretation and Radiologist Volume. Ann Surg Oncol 2012;19(12):3827–31.

97. Meltzer C, Hull M, Sundang A, et al. Association Between Annual Surgeon Total Thyroidectomy Volume and Transient and Permanent Complications. JAMA Otolaryngol Head Neck Surg 2019. https://doi.org/10.1001/jamaoto.2019.1752.

98. Quak E, Lasne Cardon A, Ciappuccini R, et al. Upfront F18-choline PET/CT versus Tc99m-sestaMIBI SPECT/CT guided surgery in primary hyperparathyroidism: the randomized phase III diagnostic trial APACH2. BMC Endocr Disord 2021;21(1):3.

99. Kim Y, Kim SW, Lee KD, et al. Real-time localization of the parathyroid gland in surgical field using Raspberry Pi during thyroidectomy: a preliminary report. Biomed Opt Express 2018;9(7):3391–8.

100. Sosa JA, Hanna JW, Robinson KA, et al. Increases in thyroid nodule fine-needle aspirations, operations, and diagnoses of thyroid cancer in the United States. Surgery 2013;154(6):1420–6 [discussion; 1426-1427].

101. Kim SM, Shu AD, Long J, et al. Declining Rates of Inpatient Parathyroidectomy for Primary Hyperparathyroidism in the US. PLoS One 2016;11(8):e0161192.

102. Lim H, Devesa SS, Sosa JA, et al. Trends in Thyroid Cancer Incidence and Mortality in the United States, 1974-2013. JAMA 2017;317(13):1338–48.

Molecular and Anatomic Imaging of Neuroendocrine Tumors

Laszlo Szidonya, MD, PhD[a,b], Eunkyung Angela Park, MD, PhD[c],
Jennifer J. Kwak, MD[d], Nadine Mallak, MD[a,*]

KEYWORDS

- Neuroendocrine tumor • Somatostatin receptor • Positron emission tomography
- Imaging • Peptide receptor radionuclide therapy • Appropriate use • Management

KEY POINTS

- Computed tomography and magnetic resonance imaging obtained for a known or suspected neuroendocrine tumor should include multiphase contrast-enhanced imaging of the abdomen.
- ^{64}Cu-DOTATATE is considered equivalent to ^{68}Ga-labelled agents; it offers logistical advantages of remote production of the radiopharmaceutical and flexible scanning times.
- High-grade neuroendocrine tumors demonstrate FDG uptake, usually with a concomitant decrease in somatostatin receptor expression. FDG uptake is an important negative prognostic factor.
- Changes in standardized uptake values alone on somatostatin receptor positron emission tomography after peptide receptor radionuclide therapy should not be interpreted as disease response or progression. The changes in size on anatomic imaging and appearance or resolution of lesions on somatostatin receptor positron emission tomography should be used instead.

INTRODUCTION

Neuroendocrine neoplasms (NENs) are a diverse group of tumors originating from neuroendocrine cells present throughout the body.[1] These tumors share common morphologic, histologic, and biochemical features; the majority express somatostatin receptors (SSTRs) on the cell surface, which can be used as imaging and therapeutic targets.[2]

[a] Oregon Health & Science University, 3181 Southwest Sam Jackson Park Road, Mail Code L340, Portland, OR 97239, USA; [b] Diagnostic Radiology, Heart and Vascular Center, Semmelweis University, Budapest, Hungary; [c] Division of Nuclear Medicine, Department of Radiology, University of Iowa Hospitals and Clinics, 200 Hawkins Drive, Iowa City, IA 52242, USA; [d] Department of Radiology, School of Medicine, University of Colorado, 12401 East 17th Avenue, Mail Stop L954, Aurora, CO 80045, USA
* Corresponding author.
E-mail address: mallak@ohsu.edu

Surg Oncol Clin N Am 31 (2022) 649–671
https://doi.org/10.1016/j.soc.2022.06.009
1055-3207/22/© 2022 Elsevier Inc. All rights reserved.

surgonc.theclinics.com

NENs include the well-differentiated neuroendocrine tumors (NETs) and the poorly differentiated neuroendocrine carcinomas (NECs). These tumors are classified based on their proliferation index (or Ki-67) and mitotic count. The 2010 and 2017 World Health Organization (WHO) classifications are detailed in **Table 1**. The most important change brought by the 2017 classification for pancreatic NETs (PNETs) is further dividing G3 tumors into well-differentiated G3 NETs (Ki-67 > 20%, however, <50%–55% typically) and NECs (high-grade by definition, with poorly differentiated morphology and Ki-67 > 20%, most commonly ≥50%–55%). NECs display more malignant features and biological behavior and include the small-cell and large-cell types.[3] In 2018, the International Agency for Research on Cancer and WHO expert consensus proposal expanded the 2017 WHO classification of PNETs to NETs of the gastrointestinal (GI) tract,[3] a change that has been reflected in the 2019 WHO classification of tumors of the digestive system.[4]

Anatomic Imaging

NETs are often discovered incidentally on computed tomography (CT) scans performed for other indications. Whenever a CT or a magnetic resonance imaging (MRI) is obtained for a known or suspected NET, it should be performed with multiphase contrast-enhanced imaging of the abdomen. Most primary PNETs and hepatic metastases are hyperenhancing and better visualized on the arterial phase (**Figs. 1 and 2**); however, due to tumor heterogeneity, even within the same individual, some tumors may be hypoenhancing and better detected on standard portal venous or delayed phases (see **Fig. 2; Fig. 3**).[5–7]

CT detection rate of primary PNETs is high, estimated at 80% to 100%[8] but it is much lower for primary small bowel NETs, reported to be around 50%.[5,9]

MRI is superior to CT for the detection of hepatic metastases.[10,11] Two particularly helpful sequences are diffusion-weighted imaging,[12] and delayed postcontrast phase using hepatospecific contrast agent (or Gadoxetic acid), which is considered the most sensitive tool for the detection of hepatic metastases.[12–14]

Several imaging features on CT and MRI have been associated with a high-tumor grade: large tumor size (>2 cm), ill-defined tumor margins, low arterial hyperenhancement, presence of pancreatic duct dilatation, nonbright T2 signal, and most importantly, high diffusion restriction on MRI.[15]

Table 1
Comparison of the 2010 and 2017 World Health Organization classifications for grading neuroendocrine neoplasms of the gastrointestinal (GI) tract and pancreas

Classification/Grade	2010		2017 (Pancreas, Later Expanded to GI Tract in 2019)	
	Mitotic Rate[a]	Ki-67%	Mitotic Rate[b]	Ki-67%
G1 (Low grade)	<2	≤2%	<2	<3%
G2 (Intermediate grade)	2–20	3%–20%	2–20	3%–20%
G3 (High grade)	>20	>20%	Well-differentiated NETs	
			>20	>20%, typically <50%–55%
			Poorly differentiated NECs	
			>20	>20%, typically ≥50%–55%

[a] Per 10 HPF.
[b] Per 2 mm².

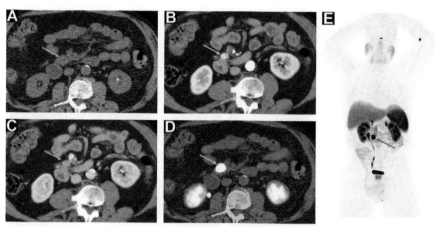

Fig. 1. PNET (*arrows*) on multiphase contrast-enhanced CT of the abdomen: precontrast (*A*), arterial (*B*), and portal venous (*C*) phases, demonstrating arterial hyperenhancement with subsequent washout. ^{64}Cu-DOTATATE PET/CT axial fused (*D*) and maximum intensity projection (MIP) (*E*) images show intense uptake in the lesion and no evidence of metastatic disease.

Functional Imaging with Somatostatin Receptor Positron Emission Tomography Agents

The SSTR expression on most NETs makes functional imaging with SSTR ligands possible.[16]

The gamma camera imaging agent ^{111}In-pentetreotide (OctreoScanTM, Curium US LLC, Maryland Heights, MO, USA) was the first Food and Drug Administration (FDA)-approved radiotracer for the functional imaging of NENs in 1994 but it has been

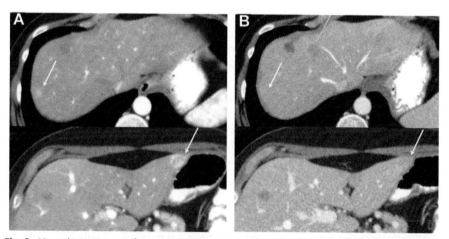

Fig. 2. Hepatic metastases from G2 PNET. Multiphase contrast enhanced CT, arterial (*A*) and portal venous (*B*) phases. Some lesions are arterially enhancing and seen only on the arterial phase (*yellow arrows*), others are hypoenhancing and better visualized on the venous phase (*green arrows*).

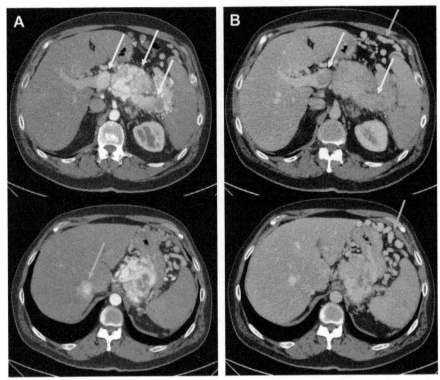

Fig. 3. G3 NET of the pancreatic tail, patient presenting with gastrointestinal bleed. Multiphase contrast-enhanced CT of the abdomen, arterial (*A*) and portal venous (*B*) phases. The mass enhances on the arterial phase, with a tumor thrombus involving the splenic and portal veins (*yellow arrows*), and collateral veins in the left abdomen (*green arrows*). Hyperenhancing liver metastasis is seen only on the arterial phase (*blue arrow*).

replaced by PET imaging agents, which are superior on all levels, as detailed in **Table 2 (Fig. 4)**.[15]

Although there are some differences in the relative affinity of the different ^{68}Ga-labelled PET radiotracers to each subtype of SSTRs, they are considered clinically equivalent:

- ^{68}Ga-DOTATATE (NETSPOT™, Advanced Accelerator Applications USA, Inc. Millburn, NJ): FDA-approved in 2016[17] and commercially available.
- ^{68}Ga-DOTATOC: FDA-approved in 2019[18] but not commercially available.
- ^{68}Ga-DOTANOC: not FDA approved yet.

In 2020, ^{64}Cu-DOTATATE (Detectnet™, Curium US LLC, Maryland Heights, MO, USA) joined the list of FDA-approved and commercially available PET radiopharmaceuticals[19] (detailed in later discussion).

A multidisciplinary group convened by the Society of Nuclear Medicine and Molecular Imaging (SNMMI) developed appropriate use criteria (AUC) for these agents, published in 2018.[20] The most appropriate indications are detailed in **Table 3** (see **Fig. 1**; **Figs. 5–10**).

In November 2020, an update to the AUC was published, adding ^{64}Cu-DOTATATE to the list of accepted SSTR PET radiopharmaceuticals, along with a new appropriate

Table 2
Comparison between the commercially available NET imaging agents

	^{111}In-pentetreotide Scan	^{68}Ga-DOTATATE PET	^{64}Cu-DOTATATE PET
Brand name	OctreoScan	NETSPOT	Detectnet
Diagnostic accuracy	Good	Significantly superior to OctreoScan for detection of small lesions (particularly lung and bone)	Slightly more superior to ^{68}Ga agents for detection of small lesions (particularly lymph nodes)
Patient convenience	Two-day protocol (imaging @ 4 and 24 or 24 and 48 h postinjection [p.i.])	One-day protocol (imaging @ 40–90 min p.i.)	One-day protocol with more flexible uptake period (imaging @ 45–180 min p.i.)
Physical T1/2	67.3 h	1.1 h	12.7 h
Injection dose	111/222 MBq (planar/SPECT)	2 MBq/kg, up to 200 MBq	148 MBq
Radiation dose[a]	Higher (13 mSV/111 MBq 26 mSv/222 MBq)	Lower (3.15 mSv/150 MBq)	Lower (4.7 mSv/148 MBq)
Availability	Readily available	Commercially available in most areas but can be limited by ^{68}Ge/^{68}Ga generator availability	Commercially available as ready-made vials, can be distributed to centers without cyclotrons

[a] Excluding radiation from low-dose CT (CTs of SPECT/CT or PET/CT).

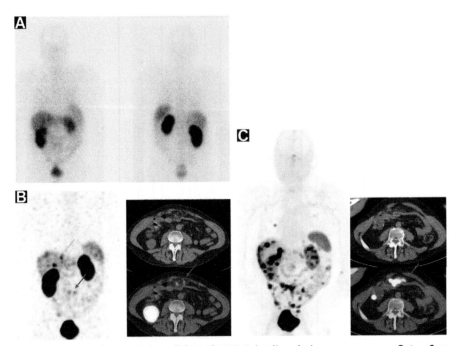

Fig. 4. Patient with resected small bowel NET. Faint liver lesions are seen on OctreoScan planar images (*A*) at 24 hours, more visible on SPECT/CT (*B, yellow arrow*), with additional peritoneal disease (*red arrows*). ^{68}Ga-DOTATATE PET/CT (*C*) shows much more extensive liver and peritoneal metastases (*red arrow*) and 2 rib lesions.

indication, which is the restaging of patients after PRRT.[21] The update also indicates that the number of SSTR PET scans performed during a patient's lifetime should not be limited, since SSTR PET plays an important role in disease management at various times. In a patient with stable disease on anatomic imaging, SSTR PET may be helpful every 2 to 3 years, to ensure that there is no disease progression with lesions occult on CT or MRI.

Pitfalls in Somatostatin Receptor Positron Emission Tomography Interpretation

Recognizing the physiologic distribution of the radiopharmaceutical and potential false positives and false negatives is crucial for an accurate interpretation of the scan.

A common pitfall is the physiologic uptake in normal or hypertrophic pancreatic islet cells, which can demonstrate focal uptake, most commonly present in the uncinate process (see **Fig. 5**) but can also be seen elsewhere in the pancreas, such as the pancreatic tail.[22,23] Generally, a higher degree of uptake is seen in NETs relative to the physiologic uptake in islet cells[24–26] but standardized uptake values (SUVs) overlap and there is no clear cutoff. Imaging features that can help differentiate include the ill-defined margins of the physiologic uptake, the curvilinear appearance when located in the uncinate process,[27] and most importantly, the absence of corresponding lesion on multiphase contrast-enhanced anatomic imaging.

Another frequent pitfall is physiologic uptake in splenic tissue. Heterotopic intrapancreatic accessory spleen (splenule) can mimic NET on CT or MRI. In fact, splenules can be found anywhere in the abdomen and can be misdiagnosed as metastatic lymph nodes or implants. It is important to recognize that SSTR PET is not an

Table 3
Most appropriate indications for somatostatin receptor PET, based on the appropriate use criteria published by the Society of Nuclear Medicine and Molecular Imaging

Indication	Comments
Initial staging after histologic diagnosis of NETs	SSTR PET is superior to both conventional imaging (CI) and SSTR scintigraphy, making it the modality of choice for staging (see **Figs. 1** and **5**)
Localization of unknown primary tumor in patients with known metastatic disease	Even when metastatic, localization of the primary site is important to guide treatment. SSTR PET helps localize the primary in patients who are left with unknown primaries after initial workup (see **Figs. 6** and **7**)
Selection of patients for SSTR-targeted peptide receptor radionuclide therapy (PRRT)	Eligibility for PRRT is determined by translating the Krenning score to the maximal intensity projection image from SSTR PET
Staging of NETs before planned surgery	Cytoreduction or surgical debulking, although noncurative, helps improve survival for patients with metastatic disease predominantly to the liver and abdominal lymph nodes. SSTR PET allows evaluation of nonresectable extrahepatic disease (most commonly to bones), which when extensive, may reduce the benefits of cytoreduction
Evaluation of mass suggestive of NET but not amenable to endoscopic or percutaneous biopsy	For example, mesenteric mass or ileal lesion
Monitoring of disease seen predominantly on SSTR PET	Osseous lesions in particular are frequently occult on CT, making SSTR PET useful for routine follow-up (see **Fig. 8**)
Evaluation of patients with biochemical evidence and symptoms of NET but without evidence on anatomic imaging and prior histologic diagnosis of NET	Although the yield is low, SSTR PET is nonetheless cost-effective, as a negative scan could prevent further diagnostic workup
Restaging at time of clinical or biochemical progression, without evidence of progression on anatomic imaging	It is very important to keep in mind the superiority of SSTR PET to CI in such scenarios: A lesion seen for the first time on SSTR PET, and is occult on CI, remains of unknown chronicity, and does not indicate disease progression. Similarly, comparison between ^{64}Cu-DOTATATE and ^{68}Ga-DOTATATE PET requires careful consideration to differentiate between true new lesions vs better visualization of preexisting ones (see **Fig. 14**)
New indeterminate lesion on anatomic imaging, with unclear progression	SSTR PET may be useful both to verify that a new lesion is a NET (in case of uptake) or raise the suspicion of tumor dedifferentiation (in case of decreasing or low uptake)

(continued on next page)

Table 3 (continued)	
Indication	**Comments**
Restaging of patients post-PRRT	(added in the updated AUC in 2020) SSTR PET serves as a new baseline. Caution not to use changes in SUV as an indicator for disease response or progression. Appearance of new lesions or resolution of preexisting lesions should be used instead (see **Figs. 9** and **10**)

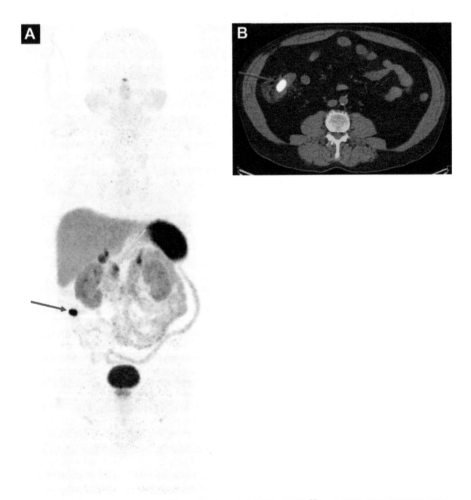

Fig. 5. Initial staging, patient with G1 ileal NET (Ki-67 < 3%). ^{68}Ga-DOTATATE PET/CT MIP image (*A*), and transaxial fused image (*B*) showing the primary tumor in the terminal ileum (*red arrow*) and no evidence of metastatic disease. Note the classic physiologic uptake in the uncinate process (*yellow arrow*).

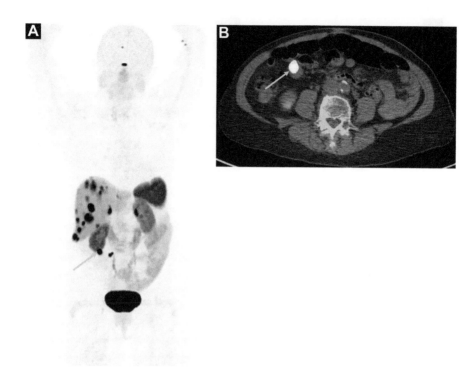

Fig. 6. Patient with hepatic lesions, biopsy proven G2 NET metastases with Ki-67 of 4%, of unknown primary. ^{64}Cu-DOTATATE PET MIP (*A*) and fused transaxial images (*B*) show intense uptake in the liver metastases, and localize the primary NET in the small bowel (*arrow*).

appropriate test to differentiate NET from a splenule, as both entities show intense uptake on this scan.[28] ^{99m}Tc-heat damaged red blood cells or ^{99m}Tc-sulfur colloid Single Photon Emission Computed Tomography (SPECT)/CT can help differentiate because splenic tissue shows uptake with these 2 agents, whereas NETs do not (**Fig. 11**).[29,30] Alternatively, MRI with superparamagnetic iron oxide (Ferumoxytol) can be used to differentiate, if available.[31]

Meningiomas demonstrate intense uptake and are frequently detected on SSTR PET as an incidental finding. Additional potential pitfalls include osteoblastic activity (degenerative bone changes, fibrous dysplasia, healing fractures, and vertebral hemangiomas) and inflammatory processes (reactive lymph nodes, infection); however, lower level of uptake can help differentiate these benign lesions from NETs (**Fig. 12**).[27]

Comparison Between ^{64}Cu-DOTATATE and ^{68}Ga-DOTATATE/TOC

The physiologic distribution of ^{64}Cu-DOTATATE (Detectnet) is similar to that of ^{68}Ga-DOTATATE, except for less splenic uptake with ^{64}Cu-DOTATATE (**Fig. 13**). The longer half-life allows production in a central location and distribution to local PET centers,[32] as well as more flexible uptake times, with no significant differences in the number of lesions detected between 60 minutes and 180 minutes postinjection scans.[33] The positron fraction of ^{64}Cu is only 18% (vs 89% for ^{68}Ga), which means fewer photon counts are collected per minute for the same injected activity, necessitating optimization of scanning parameters and protocols based on capabilities of various PET scanners. **Table 4** shows comparison of physical properties of ^{64}Cu and ^{68}Ga pertinent to PET imaging.

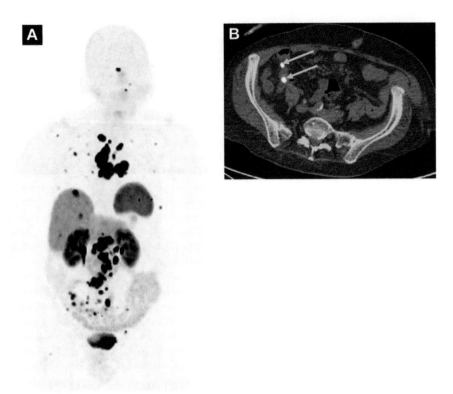

Fig. 7. ^{64}Cu-DOTATATE PET performed for localization of unknown primary in a patient with metastatic G1 NET, with liver, osseous, and lymph node metastases seen on MIP (*A*) Axial fused images (*B*) show multifocal small bowel foci of uptake (*arrows*) representing multi-focal primaries, which can be seen in 30% to 40% of small bowel NETs.

^{64}Cu-DOTATATE PET imaging is highly accurate in detecting NETs. A prospective study with 63 subjects demonstrated 91% sensitivity, 97% specificity, 97% positive predictive value, and 90% negative predictive value.[34] Excellent diagnostic performance of ^{64}Cu-DOTATATE is comparable to that of ^{68}Ga-DOTATATE/TOC. A head-to-head comparison study of ^{64}Cu-DOTATATE and ^{68}Ga-DOTATOC in 51 patients with NETs (mostly G1 and G2 gastroenteropancreatic [GEP] NETs) reported 100% sensitivity and 90% specificity for both agents, with no difference on a patient basis. However, significantly more true positive lesions were detected by ^{64}Cu-DOTATATE.[35] The higher rate of detection was mostly in small-sized lesions, presumably due to the shorter positron range of ^{64}Cu that provides better spatial resolution (**Fig. 14**, see **Table 4**).

In conclusion, ^{64}Cu-DOTATATE is a safe and high-quality radioligand for NET imaging, overall considered equivalent to ^{68}Ga-labelled agents; however, due to its unique physical properties, it requires optimization of imaging protocols and reconstruction parameters. It provides logistic advantages for PET centers without access to ^{68}Ga-labelled agents.

Fluorodeoxyglucose Positron Emission Tomography in the Imaging of Neuroendocrine Tumors

FDG PET uses a radiolabeled glucose analog that detects rapidly growing metabolically active tumors. GEP NETs demonstrate a "flip-flop" phenomenon in which low

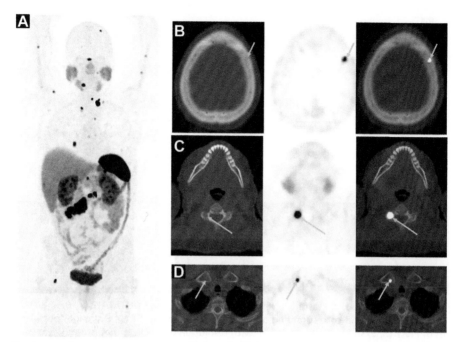

Fig. 8. Initial staging of patient with G1 small bowel NET (Ki-67 < 3%). ^{64}Cu-DOTATATE PET-CT MIP image (*A*) shows diffuse osseous metastases. Transaxial images (*B–D*) show most osseous metastases to be occult on CT (*arrows*).

uptake on FDG PET and high uptake on SSTR imaging characterize low-grade NETs (**Fig. 15**), whereas more aggressive NETs demonstrate high uptake on FDG PET and low uptake on SSTR imaging (**Fig. 16**).[36] Although most current North American consensus guidelines for the management of NETs do not mention the use of FDG

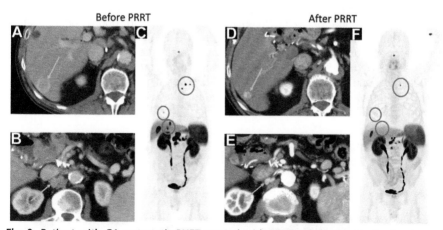

Fig. 9. Patient with G1 metastatic PNET treated with PRRT. Pretherapy contrast-enhanced abdominal CT (*A, B*) and ^{68}Ga-DOTATATE PET (*C*) show liver, retroperitoneal, and osseous metastases (*arrows*). Post-4 cycles of PRRT, decreased size of the liver metastases and retroperitoneal nodes on CT (*D, E*) (*arrows*), and resolution of several osseous and liver metastases on ^{64}Cu-DOTATATE PET (*F*) (*blue circles*). Findings consistent with disease response.

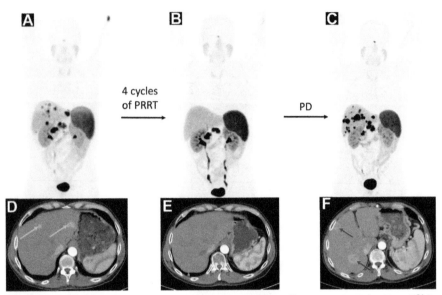

Fig. 10. Patient with G2 metastatic PNET treated with PRRT. ^{68}Ga-DOTATATE (*A, B*) and ^{64}Cu-DOTATATE (*C*) PET and corresponding arterial phase abdominal CT (*D–F*). Images post-4 cycles of PRRT (*B, E*) show disease response with resolution of the liver metastases (*yellow arrows*) compared with pretherapy scans (*A, D*). Twenty-three months later, restaging scans (*C, F*) show disease progression with multiple new liver lesions (*red arrows*).

PET, there is growing recognition that FDG PET should be considered in the evaluation of G3 tumors and more aggressive G2 tumors (Ki-67 index between 10% and 20%) as reflected in the recent European consensus guidelines.[37] In addition, there is mounting evidence that FDG PET may be a better prognosticating tool than the currently adopted histologic grading system based on the Ki-67 index for low-grade and intermediate-grade NETs (G1 and G2).[38–42]

As discussed above, within the high-grade group (Ki-67 > 20%), there exists a "mixed grade" range of well-differentiated G3 tumors to poorly differentiated NECs.[43] This results in variability of uptake on FDG PET and SSTR imaging within this heterogeneous group. Poorly differentiated carcinomas would be expected to have less SSTR and high glucose metabolic activity, thus no or little uptake on SSTR imaging and high uptake on FDG PET. However, high-grade well-differentiated G3 NETs and more aggressive intermediate-grade G2 NETs can demonstrate uptake on both FDG PET and SSTR imaging (**Fig. 17**).[38,39,41,44–46] In this group, uptake on

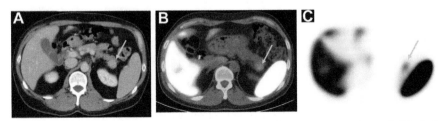

Fig. 11. Enhancing lesion in the pancreatic tail (*arrow*) on contrast-enhanced CT of the abdomen (*A*). ^{99m}Tc-heat denatured RBC scan, fused transaxial SPECT/CT (*B*) and SPECT only images (*C*) show uptake in the lesion confirming splenule.

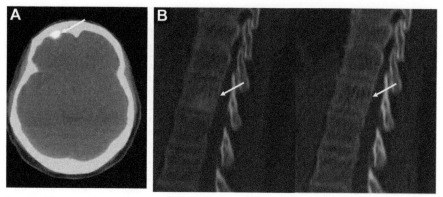

Fig. 12. (A) Arrow points to focal ^{68}Ga-DOTATATE uptake in the right frontal bone, corresponding to a benign meningioma. (B) Arrow points to mild focal ^{68}Ga-DOTATATE uptake in a vertebral body lesion, with a classic "corduroy" appearance on CT, consistent with a benign hemangioma.

SSTR imaging supports treatment with PRRT. However, FDG uptake in NETs demonstrating SSTR activity has been associated with less favorable overall survival (OS) and progression free survival (PFS) after PRRT than NETs with no FDG uptake.[39,47] It has been recommended that patients with G3 and more aggressive G2 NETs undergo

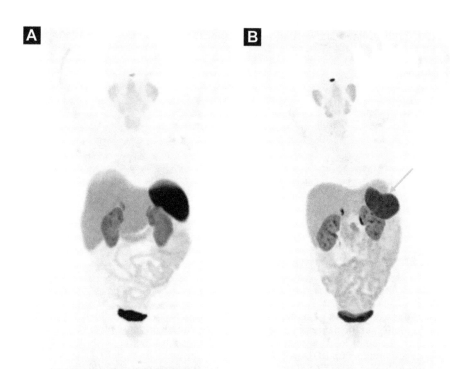

Fig. 13. Physiologic distribution of ^{68}Ga-DOTATATE (A) and ^{64}Cu-DOTATATE (B), with less intense splenic uptake (*arrow*) on the latter.

Table 4
Comparison of physical properties of ^{64}Cu and ^{68}Ga and their implications

	^{64}Cu	^{68}Ga	Implication
Half-life	12.7 h	1.1 h	^{64}Cu allows for more flexible scanning time and for remote production in central locations with delivery to each site
Positron energy (maximum)	0.65 MeV	1.90 MeV	^{64}Cu offers higher spatial resolution, which improves detection of small lesions
Positron range (mean)	0.56 mm	3.50 mm	
Production	Cyclotron	Generator/Cyclotron	
Positron fraction	18%	89%	Low signal-to-noise ratio with ^{64}Cu can be overcome by scanning longer and using noise-reducing reconstruction algorithms

"complementary" FDG PET and SSTR imaging to determine if PRRT is an appropriate treatment choice and to gauge prognosis of response to PRRT.[37]

FDG PET has also been recommended in low-grade NETs with rapid progression or with disease seen on CT/MRI with negative SSTR imaging (**Fig. 18**).[37] Otherwise, utilization of FDG PET in this group is not routinely recommended due to the slow growth and low metabolic activity. These tumors demonstrate high uptake on SSTR imaging. However, studies have shown that 49% of patients with G1/G2 tumors (and even

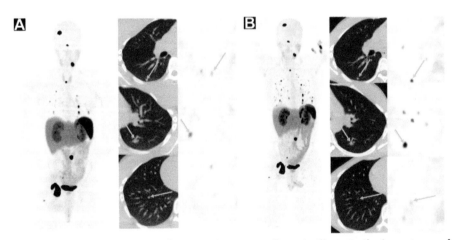

Fig. 14. We are using this case of metastatic paraganglioma to illustrate the importance of not relying solely on the degree of uptake to evaluate disease response post-PRRT, which in this case, might be at least partially related to difference in physical properties between ^{68}Ga and ^{64}Cu. Initial ^{68}Ga-DOTATATE PET/CT (*A*) and post-4 cycles of PRRT ^{64}Cu-DOTATATE PET/CT (*B*): Although more foci of uptake are seen in the lungs post-PRRT (*B*), the CT correlate shows all nodules to be stable or mildly decreased in size compared with (*A*), no new or enlarging nodules; findings consistent with overall stable disease. The better spatial resolution of ^{64}Cu can improve the detection of small lesions.

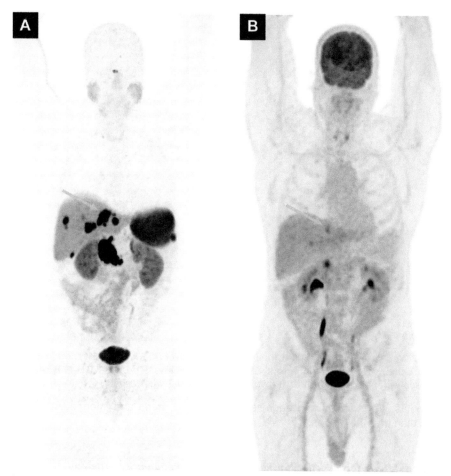

Fig. 15. G2 PNET (Ki-67 4%) metastatic to the liver (*arrows*), demonstrating high SSTR expression on ^{64}Cu-DOTATATE PET (*A*) and minimal uptake on ^{18}F-FDG PET (*B*). Studies performed 23 days apart.

21%–40% with G1 disease) can have FDG uptake, which is associated with a worse prognosis.[38–40] This paradox may be explained by biopsy sampling error, tumor heterogeneity, and Ki-67 grading observer intervariability during initial evaluation as well as tumor progression during the disease course.[48,49] There may also be unknown tumor characteristics that could promote tumor aggressiveness. The clinical relevance of FDG uptake in these tumors has been demonstrated in a recent prospective 10-year follow-up study, which demonstrated a significantly longer 5-year OS (79% vs 35%) and PFS (49% vs 18%) in patients with negative FDG PET compared with positive FDG PET, also seen in a separate subanalysis of patients with G1 and G2 tumors.[39] This study also found that in the subset of patients who underwent PRRT, 93.5% were G1 or G2, and FDG-negative patients had longer OS.[39] This finding supports a recent large retrospective study of post-PRRT patients in which FDG uptake was an independent prognostic factor associated with decreased median OS.[47] Several studies suggest that FDG uptake may be a better prognostic marker for stratifying

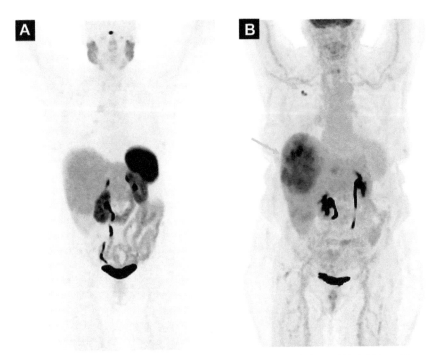

Fig. 16. Well-differentiated G2 PNET metastatic to the liver (Ki-67 10%–15%) and lungs (*arrows*), demonstrating no significant SSTR expression on ⁶⁴Cu-DOTATATE PET (*A*) and increased uptake on ¹⁸F-FDG PET (*B*). Studies performed 2 weeks apart.

the metastatic potential and aggressiveness of low-grade and intermediate-grade NETs than the Ki-67 index.[40,41,44,50]

Imaging Criteria for Selection for Peptide Receptor Radionuclide Therapy

PRRT with ¹⁷⁷Lu-DOTATATE (Lutathera™, Advanced Accelerator Applications USA, Inc., NJ) was FDA approved for the treatment of progressive metastatic well-differentiated NETs in 2018. In general, ideal candidates are patients with progressing inoperable or metastatic well-differentiated NETs who show sufficient tumor uptake on SSTR imaging, which is defined as higher-than-liver uptake.[15] Although the NETTER-1 trial (phase III trial of ¹⁷⁷Lu-DOTATATE plus long-acting octreotide versus high-dose long-acting octreotide in patients with midgut NETs),[51] which led to the FDA approval of ¹⁷⁷Lu-DOTATATE, considered patients eligible for treatment based on highest tumor uptake equal to or higher than liver based on ¹¹¹In-pentetreotide imaging,[52] it is acceptable to extrapolate this scale to SSTR PET (modified Krenning score, **Table 5**).[53] However, given the higher sensitivity of PET over planar or SPECT imaging, one should be cautious particularly for small lesions (<2 cm) because these lesions considered eligible per SSTR PET might have not shown uptake higher than liver on ¹¹¹In-pentetreotide scan.[54] In addition to the condition of a positive SSTR PET, patients should have sufficient bone marrow reserve, adequate kidney and liver function, good performance status, and expected survival longer than 3 to 6 months to be eligible for PRRT.[55] Selecting and sequencing treatments is a complex decision, and it must be based on a multidisciplinary team discussion and risk to benefit assessment of individual patients.[56]

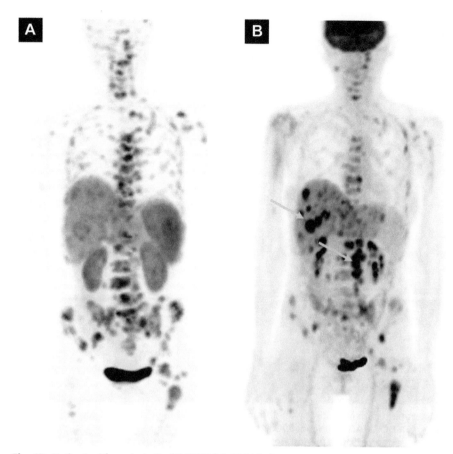

Fig. 17. Patient with metastatic G2 PNET (Ki-67 8%) demonstrating heterogeneous uptake on ^{68}Ga-DOTATATE PET (*A*) and ^{18}F-FDG PET (*B*). The bone lesions show heterogeneous uptake on both tracers; the liver and retroperitoneal nodes show uptake mostly with FDG (*arrows*).

Response Assessment Postpeptide Receptor Radionuclide Therapy

Unlike the uptake on FDG PET, which reflects tumor metabolism correlating with aggressive disease and poor prognosis, the uptake on SSTR PET reflects SSTR density on the cell surface, which carries different implications. Studies have shown that changes in the degree of uptake, that is, SUVs in NETs after PRRT do not correlate with outcomes.[57,58]

Huizing and colleagues[57] demonstrated in a retrospective analysis that the disease progression on anatomic imaging at 9 months post-PRRT indicates worse OS; however, they did not find an association between OS and the change in uptake on SSTR PET or chromogranin A levels. However, SSTR PET detected disease progression earlier than anatomic imaging, with new lesions only seen on SSTR PET but not on anatomic imaging at 3 months post-PRRT.

Tumor heterogeneity in metastatic NETs on SSTR PET has been shown to correlate with a worse prognosis and to outperform SUVs and Ki-67 as a prognostic marker.[59–61] This heterogeneity constitutes an inherent limitation for conventional

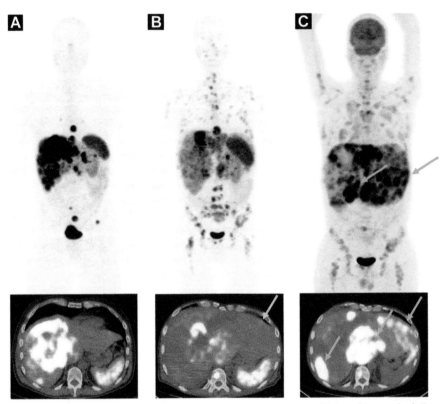

Fig. 18. Patient with metastatic well-differentiated G3 PNET. Initial (*A*) and 3 months follow-up (*B*) ⁶⁸Ga-DOTATATE MIP and fused transaxial PET/CT images show disease progression with new extensive bone metastases on (*B*); note the enlargement of the left hepatic lobe (*yellow arrow*) on (*B*) compared with (*A*) with no DOTATATE uptake, concerning for dedifferentiated/high-grade tumor, which prompted FDG PET. ¹⁸F-FDG-PET/CT (*C*) shows increased uptake in the left hepatic lobe, in addition to multiple additional hypermetabolic liver metastases (*green arrows*), compatible with high-grade lesions.

PET parameters because PRRT targets well-differentiated SSTR expressing clones, whereas sparing poorly differentiated ones.[15,62]

Although imperfect for NETs due to their slow growth, based on current literature, morphologic evaluation using Response Evaluation Criteria In Solid Tumors (RECIST 1.1),[63] which are based on changes in size of target lesions on CT/MRI, remain the most established response assessment scheme so far. SSTR PET, however, can add valuable information in determining early disease progression by detecting new

Table 5 (Modified) Kenning score	
0	No Uptake
1	Very low uptake
2	Uptake lower than or equal to liver
3	Uptake higher than liver
4	Very intense uptake or uptake higher than spleen

metastases occult on anatomic imaging[57,58] and in establishing a new post-therapy baseline scan. The SNMMI AUC emphasize that changes in SUVs alone on post-PRRT SSTR PET do not indicate disease response or progression. Response should be assessed by the disappearance of known lesions or development of new ones (see **Fig. 9**).

SUMMARY

In the last few years, SSTR PET imaging, mostly with ^{68}Ga-DOTATATE, has become the gold standard for imaging of well-differentiated NETs. SSTR PET is very useful in various clinical scenarios including but not limited to initial staging after histologic diagnosis of NETs, localizing unknown primary tumor in patients presenting with metastases, and selecting patients for PRRT. Recently, ^{64}Cu-DOTATATE was added to the list of FDA-approved radiopharmaceuticals for NET imaging. Longer half-life of ^{64}Cu expands imaging access by allowing long distance delivery and more flexible scanning windows. FDG PET complements SSTR PET, particularly for G3 and high G2 tumors. Increased FDG uptake is a significant prognostic factor implicating more aggressive disease and worse prognosis.

CLINICS CARE POINTS

- Anatomic imaging performed to evaluate NETs should include multiphase imaging of the abdomen.
- SSTR PET is the modality of choice for functional imaging of well-differentiated NETs.
- FDG PET is complimentary to SSTR PET, particularly for imaging of high grade NETs.

ACKNOWLEDGMENTS

The search tool developed by Li and colleagues[64] was invaluable in finding illustrative cases for this publication.

DISCLOSURE

The authors have nothing to disclose.

REFERENCES

1. Shah MH, Goldner WS, Benson AB, et al. Neuroendocrine and Adrenal Tumors, Version 2.2021, NCCN Clinical Practice Guidelines in Oncology. J Natl Compr Canc Netw 2021;19(7):839–68.
2. Dasari A, Shen C, Halperin D, et al. Trends in the incidence, prevalence, and survival outcomes in patients with neuroendocrine tumors in the United States. JAMA Oncol 2017;3(10):1335–42.
3. Rindi G, Klimstra DS, Abedi-Ardekani B, et al. A common classification framework for neuroendocrine neoplasms: an International Agency for Research on Cancer (IARC) and World Health Organization (WHO) expert consensus proposal. Mod Pathol Dec 2018;31(12):1770–86.
4. Nagtegaal ID, Odze RD, Klimstra D, et al. The,2019 WHO classification of tumours of the digestive system. Histopathology 2020;76(2):182–8.

5. Maxwell JE, O'Dorisio TM, Howe JR. Biochemical diagnosis and preoperative imaging of gastroenteropancreatic neuroendocrine tumors. Surg Oncol Clin N Am 2016;25(1):171–94.

6. Sahani DV, Bonaffini PA, Fernández-Del Castillo C, et al. Gastroenteropancreatic neuroendocrine tumors: role of imaging in diagnosis and management. Radiology 2013;266(1):38–61.

7. Bushnell DL, Baum RP. Standard imaging techniques for neuroendocrine tumors. Endocrinol Metab Clin North Am 2011;40(1):153–62, ix.

8. Kuo JH, Lee JA, Chabot JA. Nonfunctional pancreatic neuroendocrine tumors. Surg Clin North Am 2014;94(3):689–708.

9. Dahdaleh FS, Lorenzen A, Rajput M, et al. The value of preoperative imaging in small bowel neuroendocrine tumors. Ann Surg Oncol 2013;20(6):1912–7.

10. Dromain C, de Baere T, Lumbroso J, et al. Detection of liver metastases from endocrine tumors: a prospective comparison of somatostatin receptor scintigraphy, computed tomography, and magnetic resonance imaging. J Clin Oncol 2005;23(1):70–8.

11. Yu R, Wachsman A. Imaging of neuroendocrine tumors: indications, interpretations, limits, and pitfalls. Endocrinol Metab Clin North Am 2017;46(3):795–814.

12. Shimada K, Isoda H, Hirokawa Y, et al. Comparison of gadolinium-EOB-DTPA-enhanced and diffusion-weighted liver MRI for detection of small hepatic metastases. Eur Radiol 2010;20(11):2690–8.

13. Ba-Ssalamah A, Uffmann M, Saini S, et al. Clinical value of MRI liver-specific contrast agents: a tailored examination for a confident non-invasive diagnosis of focal liver lesions. Eur Radiol 2009;19(2):342–57.

14. Giesel FL, Kratochwil C, Mehndiratta A, et al. Comparison of neuroendocrine tumor detection and characterization using DOTATOC-PET in correlation with contrast enhanced CT and delayed contrast enhanced MRI. Eur J Radiol 2012; 81(10):2820–5.

15. Park S, Parihar AS, Bodei L, et al. Somatostatin Receptor Imaging and Theranostics: Current Practice and Future Prospects. J Nucl Med 2021;62(10):1323–9.

16. Reubi JC. Peptide receptor expression in GEP-NET. Virchows Arch 2007; 451(Suppl 1):S47–50.

17. NETSPOT (kit for the preparation of gallium Ga-68 DOTATATE injection). Available at: https://www.accessdata.fda.gov/drugsatfda_docs/nda/2016/208547Orig1s000TOC.cfm. Accessed November 27, 2021.

18. Drug approval package: Gallium DOTATOC Ga-68. 2021. Available at: https://www.accessdata.fda.gov/drugsatfda_docs/nda/2019/210828Orig1s000TOC.cfm. Accessed November 27, 2021.

19. Cu-64 DOTATATE (Detectnet™) full prescribing information. Available at: https://www.accessdata.fda.gov/drugsatfda_docs/label/2020/213227s000lbl.pdf. Accessed November 27, 2021.

20. Hope TA, Bergsland EK, Bozkurt MF, et al. Appropriate use criteria for somatostatin receptor PET imaging in neuroendocrine tumors. J Nucl Med 2018;59(1): 66–74.

21. Hope TA. Updates to the appropriate-use criteria for somatostatin receptor PET. J Nucl Med 2020;61(12):1764.

22. Jacobsson H, Larsson P, Jonsson C, et al. Normal uptake of 68Ga-DOTA-TOC by the pancreas uncinate process mimicking malignancy at somatostatin receptor PET. Clin Nucl Med 2012;37(4):362–5.

23. Delbeke D, Newman G, Deppen S, et al. 68Ga-DOTATATE: significance of uptake in the tail of the pancreas in patients without lesions. Clin Nucl Med 2019;44(11): 851–4.
24. Kroiss A, Putzer D, Decristoforo C, et al. 68Ga-DOTA-TOC uptake in neuroendocrine tumour and healthy tissue: differentiation of physiological uptake and pathological processes in PET/CT. Eur J Nucl Med Mol Imaging 2013;40(4):514–23.
25. Al-Ibraheem A, Bundschuh RA, Notni J, et al. Focal uptake of 68Ga-DOTATOC in the pancreas: pathological or physiological correlate in patients with neuroendocrine tumours? Eur J Nucl Med Mol Imaging 2011;38(11):2005–13.
26. Krausz Y, Rubinstein R, Appelbaum L, et al. Ga-68 DOTA-NOC uptake in the pancreas: pathological and physiological patterns. Clin Nucl Med 2012;37(1): 57–62.
27. Hofman MS, Lau WF, Hicks RJ. Somatostatin receptor imaging with 68Ga DOTA-TATE PET/CT: clinical utility, normal patterns, pearls, and pitfalls in interpretation. Radiographics 2015;35(2):500–16.
28. Lancellotti F, Sacco L, Cerasari S, et al. Intrapancreatic accessory spleen false positive to 68Ga-Dotatoc: case report and literature review. World J Surg Oncol 2019;17(1):117.
29. Shah M, McClelland A, Moadel R, et al. Splenule disguised as pancreatic mass: elucidated with SPECT liver-spleen scintigraphy. Clin Nucl Med 2014;39(9): e405–6.
30. Belkhir SM, Archambaud F, Prigent A, et al. Intrapancreatic accessory spleen diagnosed on radionuclide imaging. Clin Nucl Med 2009;34(9):642–4.
31. Muehler MR, Rendell VR, Bergmann LL, et al. Ferumoxytol-enhanced MR imaging for differentiating intrapancreatic splenules from other tumors. Abdom Radiol (Ny) 2021;46(5):2003–13.
32. Pfeifer A, Knigge U, Binderup T, et al. 64Cu-DOTATATE PET for neuroendocrine tumors: a prospective head-to-head comparison with 111In-DTPA-Octreotide in 112 Patients. J Nucl Med 2015;56(6):847–54.
33. Loft M, Carlsen EA, Johnbeck CB, et al. (64)Cu-DOTATATE PET in Patients with neuroendocrine neoplasms: prospective, head-to-head comparison of imaging at 1 hour and 3 hours After Injection. J Nucl Med 2021;62(1):73–80.
34. Delpassand ES, Ranganathan D, Wagh N, et al. (64)Cu-DOTATATE PET/CT for imaging patients with known or suspected somatostatin receptor-positive neuroendocrine tumors: results of the first U.S. prospective, reader-masked clinical trial. J Nucl Med 2020;61(6):890–6.
35. Johnbeck CB, Knigge U, Loft A, et al. Head-to-Head Comparison of (64)Cu-DOTATATE and (68)Ga-DOTATOC PET/CT: A Prospective Study of 59 Patients with Neuroendocrine Tumors. J Nucl Med 2017;58(3):451–7.
36. Kayani I, Bomanji JB, Groves A, et al. Functional imaging of neuroendocrine tumors with combined PET/CT using 68Ga-DOTATATE (DOTA-DPhe1,Tyr3-octreotate) and 18F-FDG. Cancer 2008;112(11):2447–55.
37. Ambrosini V, Kunikowska J, Baudin E, et al. Consensus on molecular imaging and theranostics in neuroendocrine neoplasms. Eur J Cancer Mar 2021;146:56–73.
38. Bahri H, Laurence L, Edeline J, et al. High prognostic value of 18F-FDG PET for metastatic gastroenteropancreatic neuroendocrine tumors: a long-term evaluation. J Nucl Med 2014;55(11):1786–90.
39. Binderup T, Knigge U, Johnbeck CB, et al. (18)F-FDG PET is Superior to WHO Grading as a Prognostic Tool in Neuroendocrine Neoplasms and Useful in Guiding PRRT: A Prospective 10-Year Follow-up Study. J Nucl Med 2021;62(6): 808–15.

40. Binderup T, Knigge U, Loft A, et al. 18F-fluorodeoxyglucose positron emission tomography predicts survival of patients with neuroendocrine tumors. Clin Cancer Res 2010;16(3):978–85.
41. Ezziddin S, Adler L, Sabet A, et al. Prognostic stratification of metastatic gastroenteropancreatic neuroendocrine neoplasms by 18F-FDG PET: feasibility of a metabolic grading system. J Nucl Med 2014;55(8):1260–6.
42. Rinzivillo M, Partelli S, Prosperi D, et al. Clinical Usefulness of (18)F-Fluorodeoxyglucose Positron Emission Tomography in the Diagnostic Algorithm of Advanced Entero-Pancreatic Neuroendocrine Neoplasms. Oncologist 2018; 23(2):186–92.
43. Tang LH, Untch BR, Reidy DL, et al. Well-differentiated neuroendocrine tumors with a morphologically apparent high-grade component: a pathway distinct from poorly differentiated neuroendocrine carcinomas. Clin Cancer Res 2016; 22(4):1011–7.
44. Binderup T, Knigge U, Loft A, et al. Functional imaging of neuroendocrine tumors: a head-to-head comparison of somatostatin receptor scintigraphy, 123I-MIBG scintigraphy, and 18F-FDG PET. J Nucl Med 2010;51(5):704–12.
45. Deroose CM, Hindie E, Kebebew E, et al. Molecular Imaging of Gastroenteropancreatic Neuroendocrine Tumors: Current Status and Future Directions. J Nucl Med 2016;57(12):1949–56.
46. Has Simsek D, Kuyumcu S, Turkmen C, et al. Can complementary 68Ga-DOTA-TATE and 18F-FDG PET/CT establish the missing link between histopathology and therapeutic approach in gastroenteropancreatic neuroendocrine tumors? J Nucl Med 2014;55(11):1811–7.
47. Zhang J, Liu Q, Singh A, et al. Prognostic Value of (18)F-FDG PET/CT in a Large Cohort of Patients with Advanced Metastatic Neuroendocrine Neoplasms Treated with Peptide Receptor Radionuclide Therapy. J Nucl Med 2020;61(11):1560–9.
48. Polley MY, Leung SC, McShane LM, et al. An international Ki67 reproducibility study. J Natl Cancer Inst 2013;105(24):1897–906.
49. Singh S, Hallet J, Rowsell C, et al. Variability of Ki67 labeling index in multiple neuroendocrine tumors specimens over the course of the disease. Eur J Surg Oncol 2014;40(11):1517–22.
50. Garin E, Le Jeune F, Devillers A, et al. Predictive value of 18F-FDG PET and somatostatin receptor scintigraphy in patients with metastatic endocrine tumors. J Nucl Med 2009;50(6):858–64.
51. Strosberg J, El-Haddad G, Wolin E, et al. Phase 3 Trial of (177)Lu-Dotatate for Midgut Neuroendocrine Tumors. N Engl J Med 2017;376(2):125–35.
52. Krenning EP, Valkema R, Kooij PP, et al. Scintigraphy and radionuclide therapy with [indium-111-labelled-diethyl triamine penta-acetic acid-D-Phe1]-octreotide. Ital J Gastroenterol Hepatol 1999;31(Suppl 2):S219–23.
53. Werner RA, Solnes LB, Javadi MS, et al. SSTR-RADS Version 1.0 as a Reporting System for SSTR PET Imaging and Selection of Potential PRRT Candidates: A Proposed Standardization Framework. J Nucl Med Jul 2018;59(7):1085–91.
54. Hope TA, Calais J, Zhang L, et al. (111)In-Pentetreotide Scintigraphy Versus (68) Ga-DOTATATE PET: Impact on Krenning Scores and Effect of Tumor Burden. J Nucl Med Sep 2019;60(9):1266–9.
55. Hicks RJ, Kwekkeboom DJ, Krenning E, et al. ENETS consensus guidelines for the standards of care in neuroendocrine neoplasia: peptide receptor radionuclide therapy with radiolabeled somatostatin analogues. Neuroendocrinology 2017;105(3):295–309.

56. Hope TA, Bodei L, Chan JA, et al. NANETS/SNMMI Consensus Statement on Patient Selection and Appropriate Use of (177)Lu-DOTATATE Peptide Receptor Radionuclide Therapy. J Nucl Med 2020;61(2):222-7.
57. Huizing DMV, Aalbersberg EA, Versleijen MWJ, et al. Early response assessment and prediction of overall survival after peptide receptor radionuclide therapy. Cancer Imaging 2020;20(1):57.
58. Gabriel M, Oberauer A, Dobrozemsky G, et al. 68Ga-DOTA-Tyr3-octreotide PET for assessing response to somatostatin-receptor-mediated radionuclide therapy. J Nucl Med 2009;50(9):1427-34.
59. Werner RA, Ilhan H, Lehner S, et al. Pre-therapy somatostatin receptor-based heterogeneity predicts overall survival in pancreatic neuroendocrine tumor patients undergoing peptide receptor radionuclide therapy. Mol Imaging Biol 2019;21(3):582-90.
60. Werner RA, Lapa C, Ilhan H, et al. Survival prediction in patients undergoing radionuclide therapy based on intratumoral somatostatin-receptor heterogeneity. Oncotarget 2017;8(4):7039-49.
61. Graf J, Pape UF, Jann H, et al. Prognostic Significance of somatostatin receptor heterogeneity in progressive neuroendocrine tumor treated with Lu-177 DOTA-TOC or Lu-177 DOTATATE. Eur J Nucl Med Mol Imaging 2020;47(4):881-94.
62. Roll W, Weckesser M, Seifert R, et al. Imaging and liquid biopsy in the prediction and evaluation of response to PRRT in neuroendocrine tumors: implications for patient management. Eur J Nucl Med Mol Imaging 2021;48(12):4016-27.
63. Eisenhauer EA, Therasse P, Bogaerts J, et al. New response evaluation criteria in solid tumours: revised RECIST guideline (version 1.1). Eur J Cancer 2009;45(2):228-47.
64. Li N, Maresh G, Cretcher M, et al., A modern non-SQL approach to radiology-centric search engine design with clinical validation, 2020, arXiv preprint arXiv:2007.02124.

Applications of Three-Dimensional Printing in Surgical Oncology

Catherine T. Byrd, MD[a], Natalie S. Lui, MD, MAS[a],
H. Henry Guo, MD, PhD[b,1,]*

KEYWORDS

- 3D printing • Surgical oncology • Education • Surgical planning
- Surgical simulation

KEY POINTS

- Three-dimensional (3D) printing uses data from a patient's own imaging. Relevant structures from the imaging are segmented and then printed.
- 3D printing can be a valuable resource for surgical planning in the setting of complex anatomy or unusual tumors.
- 3D printing allows trainees and providers to practice and refine surgical skills through simulation.
- 3D printing enables creation of durable tactile models incorporating biomimicry for improved understanding of basic and pathologic anatomy.
- 3D printing can be used to create patient-specific surgical guides and implants.

HISTORY OF THREE-DIMENSIONAL PRINTING

Three-dimensional (3D) printing, also referred to as additive manufacturing and rapid prototyping, involves the conversion of computer renderings to physical 3D models through deposition of material in 0.001 to 0.1-inch-thick layers, making use of a variety of substrates including plastics, metals, plaster, and naturally derived materials.[1–3] The first printing techniques involving plastic were developed in the early 1980s. The designers initially struggled to market 3D printing technology to the public.[2] The technology was first patented in 1986, when Charles Hull developed the stereolithography (SLA) process.[1,2] Hull and others continued to build on this technology, developing techniques to convert 2D images to virtual computer renderings that are produced as physical 3D models.[2] The patent on a commonly used 3D printing technology, fused deposition modeling (FDM), remained in effect until 2009.[2] After many

[a] Department of Cardiothoracic Surgery, Stanford University, Falk Building, 300 Pasteur Dr, Stanford, CA 94305, USA; [b] Department of Radiology, Stanford University, Stanford, 435 Quarry Rd, Palo Alto, CA 94304, USA
[1] Present address: 453 Quarry Road, Palo Alto, CA 94304.
* Corresponding author.
E-mail address: HENRYGUO@STANFORD.EDU

Surg Oncol Clin N Am 31 (2022) 673–684
https://doi.org/10.1016/j.soc.2022.06.005
1055-3207/22/© 2022 Elsevier Inc. All rights reserved.

3D printing technologies became open source, there was exponential growth in 3D printing, particularly in medicine.[1,2,4] To date, almost all surgical specialties have applied 3D printing to clinical practice and educational training.[5,6]

3D Printing Steps: Preprocessing, Processing, and Postprocessing

Preprocessing

The preprocessing stage involves imaging the specimen of interest and segmenting the imaging data to create a 3D rendering of the specimen to be printed.[2] Computed tomography (CT) and MRI are the leading imaging modalities of choice. Acquired imaging data are saved in digital imaging and communications in medicine format.[2] Intravenous and sometimes enteral contrast can be administered to enhance and highlight structures within the specimen.[6] Multiple scans during different phases of contrast enhancement, such as early arterial, late arterial, portal venous, and delayed phases, can be acquired. Image reconstruction through the specimen, typically in thin slices of 1 mm or less and not greater than 2 mm, allow for recreation of anatomic features and ensure precision of the subsequent model.[6]

The images are then segmented by selecting and highlighting structures within the specimen that will eventually be printed. Segmentation can be performed manually or be partially or entirely automated using nonproprietary or proprietary software.[2] Depending on the goals of the 3D print, separate structures such as organ parenchyma, nerves, vessels, or bone are included or excluded from renderings, and only desired structures remain at the end of this step.[6] Segmentations are rendered as surface meshes composed of small triangles that communicate the location, size, and shape of each structure.[2] They are expressed using standard tessellation language.[1] The technologist, surgeon, and/or radiologist evaluate and validate the 3D virtual reconstruction in preparation for 3D printing (**Fig. 1**). Areas of abnormality (eg, a sharp corner on a blood vessel) are corrected. Aspects of the rendering that do not serve the

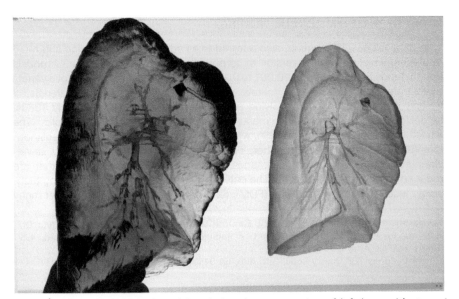

Fig. 1. Juxtaposed 3D-printed model and virtual reconstruction of left lung with stage 1 adenocarcinoma of the left upper lobe, with lung parenchyma depicted in clear plastic and cancerous nodule in red. The patient underwent successful resection.

end goal are eliminated. Decisions such as colors and materials for different structures, or ways to construct the model, such as making some parts detachable or suspended, are also made at this stage.[6]

Printing decisions are shaped by factors such as goal of the project, turnaround time, printer availability, and cost.[2] Models that will be used during surgery must be made from autoclavable materials. Implanted prostheses require biocompatible materials. Models for practicing surgical skills should exhibit biomimicry—be as similar to human tissue as possible.[2] Models that will be used to explain procedures to multiple patients must be made from durable materials.

Natural or synthetic polymers are commonly used materials.[2] Metals, ceramics, and plasters may also be used for specialized applications.[1,5] The United States Food and Drug Administration (USFDA) has approved polymers for implantation into the human body, including polycaprolactone, polylactic acid, and polylacticcoglycolic acid, with the last 2 thermoplastic materials derived from natural materials.[5] The varying properties of these polymers, such as different melting points, biodegradation profiles, and mechanical specifications, allow for these polymers to be combined in different proportions to create a final product that best suits the goals of the print.[5]

Processing

Many 3D printing technologies are available. More commonly used methods in health care include powder bed fusion, material extrusion, material jetting, and vat photopolymerization.[1,2] *Powder bed fusion* is also known as selective laser sintering (**Fig. 2**A). During this process, individual layers of powdered resin are fused by heat from a

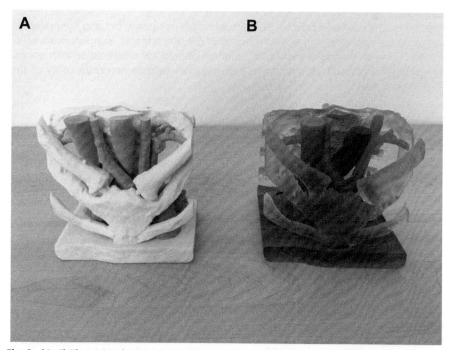

Fig. 2. (*A, B*) Thoracic inlet anatomy 3D printed using gypsum powder bed fusion (*left*) and polyjet/inkjet printing (*right*). Color conventions of the gypsum and plastic models, respectively are bone white/translucent, arteries red, veins blue, trachea gray/black.

focused CO_2 laser, leading to precise and flexible models.[1,2,5] The resin used is a thermoplastic that can be impervious to high temperatures and many chemical compounds.[2] This process and its materials can be very expensive.[2] Selective laser sintering is also used to print metal prostheses for implantation.[7,8]

Material extrusion encompasses several submethods including direct ink writing (DIW), FDM, and fused filament fabrication (FFF).[2] In DIW, a nozzle continuously layers the materials onto a stage. Different types of materials, commonly silicone, can be printed with this method. Limitations of DIW include decreased precision and higher cost when compared with other methods.[2] In FDM, beads of thermoplastic are deposited in layers from a nozzle onto the stage.[1,2] In FFF, a continuous filament of thermoplastic, most commonly polylactic acid, is deposited in a similar fashion.[2] FDM and FFF models are often less costly and more frequently used but can be restricted by limitations of available colors in a single print.[2]

Material jetting is also known as inkjet printing (**Fig. 2**B). An ink composed of the printing material is deposited in droplets in individual layers to create the print,[1] using heat via a thermal head or using acoustics via a piezoelectric head.[2] The thermal process prints quickly and at a lower cost but droplet sizes can be heterogenous.[2] The piezoelectric process can be susceptible to nozzle obstruction but droplets sizes tend to be more uniform.

Vat photopolymerization uses SLA, in which an ultraviolet laser hardens layers of liquid resin within a vat of unpolymerized material as the model is progressively built.[2] On completion, the model is removed from the vat and cured. Although the SLA process can be expensive, it is among the fastest 3D printing technologies and can produce geometrically challenging structures.[2]

Postprocessing

After the model has been printed, postprocessing is necessary to bring the project to completion. Postprocessing entails removal of printing artifacts, support material, or excess filaments. Curing of the model, addition of color, or modification with accessory components such as attachments or magnets help to maximize utility of the 3D-printed model.[2]

Three-Dimensional Printed Models Provide Unique Perspective

One of the advantages of 3D-printed models is that they allow users to understand anatomy and relationships between structures in a way that traditional imaging (CT, MR, etc.) and virtual computer renderings cannot.[4,6] Although seasoned surgeons are able to create a 3D mental picture of relevant anatomy based on imaging and operative experience, such a task can be difficult for surgeons-in-training, medical students, and patients.[9] Complex cases can challenge even the most seasoned surgeons, such as when anatomy is altered by a tumor.[9]

Three-dimensional printed models inherently provide a tactile aspect to understanding of 3D spatial relationships, using haptic perception—the ability to explore an object through touch—to further inform and improve the understanding of a structure first gained through sight. The user can feel and thus better understand the details and relationships of anatomic structures, particularly with enhanced depth perception.[6,9] The addition of touch has been shown to decrease the amount of time required to understand a structure and its relationships, as compared with relying on visual information alone.[6] Biomimicry by 3D-printed models can further enhance tactile feedback for the user.[2] Surgeons and trainees are therefore able to practice surgical skills or plan ahead for potential anatomic challenges in performing a complex procedure.[6]

Thus, proceduralists are more prepared and confident before complicated and potentially high-risk interventions.

Surgical oncologists can advance several goals using 3D-printed models:

1. Surgical planning
2. Skills refinement
3. Education of trainees and patients
4. Surgical guides
5. Implants or prostheses

Surgical Planning

Seventy-four percent of surveyed attending surgeons thought that 3D-printed models are beneficial to preoperative surgical planning.[10] Three-dimensional printed models have been used to plan colorectal cancer resection. In one case, a liver model facilitated an R0 resection in colorectal cancer liver metastasectomy.[11] In another case report, a 3D model for laparoscopic right hemicolectomy helped the surgeons better understand the regional anatomy of planned lymphadenectomy, particularly of the typically variable mesenteric vasculature.[12] The patient was able to undergo an R0 resection and 24 lymph nodes were harvested, 12 of which were positive for metastatic disease.[12]

Another beneficial application of 3D printing is in video-assisted thoracic surgery (VATS) segmentectomy of ground-glass pulmonary nodules.[13] Localization of ground-glass nodules can be difficult given their lack of tactile feedback with minimally invasive techniques. Chen and colleagues 3D-printed reconstructions of nodules with adjacent vasculature, bronchus, hilum, and lymph nodes for 51 patients.[13] Subsequent outcomes were compared with 38 control patients who underwent VATS segmentectomy without preoperative 3D printing. The 3D-printed group experienced fewer conversions to open surgery (0 vs 10.5%, $P < .05$) and fewer conversions to lobectomy (0 vs 10.5%, $P < .05$) compared with the control group. Operative times were lower (2.07 ± 0.24 hours vs 2.55 ± 0.41 hours, $P < .05$) and the estimated blood loss was halved (43.25 ± 13.63 mL vs 96.68 ± 32.82 mL, $P < .05$) as compared with the control group without the benefit of preoperative 3D-printed models.[13]

Skills Refinement

Three-dimensional-printed models allow proceduralist to practice surgical skills in a low-risk environment. Given the patient-specific nature of 3D-printed models, the surgeon can print an accurate version of the anatomy that they will encounter. Biomimicry can further enhance excellent simulation and skills training. For example, new trainees often struggle to learn the level of force to use when manipulating tissue, unfortunately often using too much force, leading to as much as 50% of surgical errors.[2] Using a 3D-printed model with similar mechanical properties can help such learners calibrate the level of force to exert.[2] Moreover, learners can repeatedly attempt and refine a specific skill.[6] One example is in the teaching of mediastinoscopy in sampling of mediastinal lymph nodes and the determination of surgical candidacy. A 3D-printed model of the mediastinum to practice mediastinoscopy was provided to surgical trainees and significantly increased their understanding of the anatomy and improved their performance of mediastinoscopy.[14]

Similarly, experienced surgeons can use 3D-printed models to prepare for complex cases or attempt a new technique, such as converting a procedure from a laparoscopic to a robotic approach, with minimal patient risk. Pugliese and colleagues have practiced nephrectomy and robotic splenic artery aneurysmectomy using 3D-printed models, and the surgeons who underwent this training reported this to be an effective mechanism to practice their skills and improve their confidence before surgeries.[6]

Education of Trainees and Patients

More than 90% of surveyed surgery residents and medical students thought that 3D-printed models improve understanding of uncomplicated anatomy or anatomy disrupted by a pathologic process.[10] Trainees also conveyed that they would appreciate incorporation of such models into formal education (**Fig. 3**).[10]

Those in the medical field at all levels of training can benefit and learn using 3D-printed models. Marconi and colleagues printed the anatomy of 15 patients undergoing either laparoscopic splenectomy, nephrectomy, or pancreatectomy.[15] They subsequently tested 10 medical students, 10 general surgeons, and 10 radiologists on their understanding of the surgical anatomy after examining the anatomy using conventional images from CT, a 3D virtual reconstruction, and a 3D-printed model. Overall, scores improved by 8% points from baseline examination with only CT images to examination using 3D virtual and printed reconstructions ($P < .001$). Additionally, all 3 groups required less time examining the 3D-printed models as compared with reviewing images from conventional CT,[15] underscoring the improvement that haptic perception adds to understanding of anatomic structure. Ninety-three percent of study participants reported 3D models to be either useful or very useful for understanding anatomy.[15]

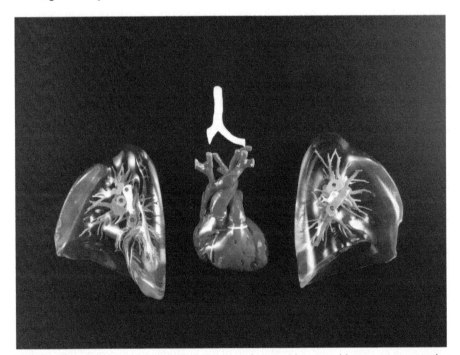

Fig. 3. Exploded view of polyjet/inkjet 3D print of normal heart and lung anatomy used at our institution for education. Color conventions are as follows: clear lung parenchyma; white airways; blue for deoxygenated blood of systemic veins, right heart, and pulmonary arteries; and red for oxygenated blood of system arteries, left heart, and pulmonary veins. Cardiac valve planes are marked in white. Magnets were added in postprocessing and the model can be reassembled or taken apart to demonstrate anatomic relationships.

Another group also found that 3D-printed models improved surgical resident learning as compared with 3D virtual reconstruction alone.[16] Surgery residents either received 3D-printed models of pancreatic tumors or reviewed 3D virtual reconstructions of the same tumors on computer displays. After instruction with either the model or virtual reconstruction, residents were then tested on their understanding of the anatomy, appropriate operative steps based on the tumor location, and response to potential complications. The residents who were provided with 3D-printed models exhibited greater understanding of the anatomy and were able to develop better surgical plans. The mean quality of surgical plan scores were significantly higher at 76.4 ± 10.5 for those provided with 3D-printed models as opposed to 66.5 ± 11.2 for residents who only reviewed virtual renderings, $P = .018$.

More than 90% of surveyed attending surgeons thought 3D-printed models would be beneficial to patient education in the office.[10] Three-dimensional printed models can be used to explain anatomy to patients preoperatively. Weinberg and colleagues used a 3D-printed rib cage chondrosarcoma model to explain an upcoming surgery to their patient.[17] The presence of the model improved understanding for the patient and did not otherwise alter the informed consent process. Per the patient, "Compared with the X-rays and scans which I found difficult to understand, the 3D-printed model allowed me to more easily appreciate what was wrong, and more importantly, I could easily relay my diagnosis onto my family and friends."[17] In another example, Yoon and colleagues reported a randomized control study in which customized 3D-printed models were used during informed consent discussions for stage I lung cancers.[18] Half of the 20 patients enrolled underwent an informed consent discussion with the use of a 3D-printed model of their lung cancer and the surrounding anatomy. The other half participated in a conventional informed consent discussion. Patients who were provided with a 3D model reported significantly higher knowledge scores on a Likert scale questionnaire ($P = .02$).[18]

Surgical Guides

Customized 3D-printed surgical guides have played key roles in the treatment of malignancies,[4] including an increasing role in lung nodule tissue sampling and subsequent pathologic cancer diagnosis. The introduction of low-dose CT screening for current and recent former smokers has led to an increased detection of small but suspicious lung nodules that often measure less than 2 cm.[20] Current standard of care for further workup includes CT-guided percutaneous localization and biopsy of such nodules. Although CT-guided biopsy is successful in up to 95% of cases, intraprocedural radiation dose and multiple insertions of hookwire(s) during the localization process leading to potential complications such as hemothorax or pneumothorax are concerns.[19,20] Three-dimensional printed navigational templates were thus designed to potentially improve this process. Using a preprocedural CT, a 3D-printed template customized to the patient's anatomy and nodule location was designed and printed using SLA. A noninferiority trial with 190 patients compared outcomes using the 3D-printed template versus conventional CT-guided approach.[21] Localization with the template was faster than with conventional localization (7.4 vs 9.5 minutes, $P < .001$). Using the 3D-printed template, fewer hookwire insertions were required as compared with conventional localization, with only one required insertion in 89% of cases using the templated approach as compared with only 6% of cases using convention localization, in which 94% of cases required 2 or more insertions ($P < .001$). Additionally, patients who benefited from the 3D-printed template were exposed to less intraprocedural radiation than those who underwent conventional localization (229 vs 313 mGy, $P < .001$).[21]

Three-dimensional printing has been used in reconstruction of the bony structures in head and neck cancers requiring segmental mandibulectomy.[22] A 3D-printed model of a patient's mandible as it would seem after planned resection was printed preoperatively, allowing for titanium screw plates that are usually molded to the mandible intraoperatively to be preshaped to the 3D-printed model and sterilized preoperatively. The group also created 3D-printed cutting guides for the fibular free flap used to reconstruct the mandible, which avoided blood vessel perforators in this location. Overall, these techniques saved 2.0 to 2.5 hours of operative time and were associated with improved free flap survival.[22]

Implants or Prostheses

Locally advanced lung cancer or breast cancer involving the chest wall require en bloc resections of the tumor and chest wall, with mortality for those who require concomitant chest wall resection up to 3 times higher than those who do not require chest wall resection, in part due to negative effects on respiratory mechanics.[23] Thus, one group used 3D printing to create custom chest wall prostheses for 3 patients.[23] Several ribs were printed for 2 patients and a sternum printed for another patient. The prints were used to create silicone molds, which were sterilized and used to form implantable prostheses from methyl methacrylate. There were neither associated complications, increased length of stay, nor an increased 30-day mortality associated with implantations of the custom chest wall prostheses. Average cost of creating the prostheses at approximately US$44 was much lower than a conventional cadaveric or titanium implant.[23]

Patient-unique 3D-printed titanium-based chest wall implants have also been constructed, as described by Goldsmith and coworkers in a patient with chondrosarcoma.[8] Using 3D virtual reconstructions from the patient's CT, resection of the right second to fourth ribs and hemisternum was planned, allowing for appropriate resection margins. The group printed custom cutting guides and a personalized titanium implant with engineered suture holes to replace the resected hemichest wall, which was covered with a latissimus dorsi flap. The patient has not experienced complications with the implant or reoccurrence of tumor 18 months after surgery.[8]

Additional Advantages of Three-Dimensional Printing in Medicine

Multiple potential advantages of using 3D printing in surgical oncology include decreased operative time, decreased blood loss, reduced radiation exposure, and improved surgical outcomes.[4,13,20–22,24] Of 145 studies reviewed by Tack and colleagues that evaluated the effect of 3D-printed models on operative time, 123 (85%) reported a decrease in operative times.[4] Chen and colleagues demonstrated an overall decrease in estimated blood loss when 3D-printed models were used for preoperative surgical planning,[13] which can facilitate the identification of avascular planes to operate and help localize a lesion more quickly, leading to decreased intraoperative exploration and associated potential for complications.[4,6]

As demonstrated by Zhang and coworkers, the use of a 3D-printed navigational template for CT-guided lung nodule localization resulted in a significant decrease in radiation dose, with an average of one less CT pass per lesion.[20,21] In the systematic review by Tack and colleagues, 17 studies found a decrease in radiation exposure, 3 found equivalent radiation exposure as compared with conventional techniques, and 9 found an increase in radiation exposure.[4]

Finally, clinical outcomes were more frequently improved with 3D-printed model use as compared with conventional techniques. Of the 243 studies reviewed by Tack and colleagues, 195 (80%) demonstrated improved outcomes.[4] Three-dimensional-printed models were also associated with higher levels of "surgical accuracy."[24]

Concerns About Three-Dimensional Printing in Surgical Oncology

As with any developing technology, several aspects of 3D-printed models raise potential for concern and would benefit from further improvement. Three-dimensional printing is still not able to achieve perfect biomimicry, which is important for highly realistic practice of surgical skills. Currently no 3D-printed material, including natural polymers such as alginate or gelatin, can perfectly mimic mechanical properties of in vivo tissue.[2] In the authors' experience, synthetic thermoplastics, although flexible, exhibit nonphysiological resistance when inserting and removing surgical instruments, decreasing the level of realism of a surgical simulation. In terms of personalized prostheses, the number and types of USFDA approved implantable 3D-printed materials are still limited, and those that do exist lack biomimicry,[5] hindering wider use of 3D-printed implants.

Turnaround time has been an ongoing concern for 3D printing in surgical planning. On the low end, some articles describe the production of custom 3D models, from segmentation to postprocessed print, in as little as 8 hours.[19,21] Others have described up to 160 hours to prepare a 3D-printed model.[11] Variation stems from multiple factors such as availability of personnel, institutional experience, complexity of anatomy and segmentation, size, shipping speed if outsourced, and the 3D printing technology being used. Processing times for lower priority models, such as for education, can take even longer, given the preferential allocation of resources for time-sensitive clinical applications and iterative approaches often necessary to optimize designs for realism and deeper understanding.

The cost of 3D-printed models can be variable, and at times nebulous. Although the costs of materials to print models are often reported in published studies, the additional time investment by physicians and technologists for segmentation, design, and model colors and materials selection are often not accounted for. It is anticipated that in addition to improved surgical and patient outcomes, investments in 3D printing may lead to cost savings by facilitating shorter operating times and decreased rate of complications. With wider adoption and economies of scale, 3D printing costs continue to decrease. In the early days of medical 3D printing, 2010 to 2012, model printing costs were in the range of US\$1200 to \$4000.[10] In contrast, more recent prices range from US\$44 to \$226.[11,15,19,20,23] Although such estimates typically do not include the overhead costs required to purchase and site a 3D printer or the associated labor costs. The learning curve and investment to develop an institutional 3D printing program can be steep.[5] Although potentially cost-saving business models such as outsourcing of design and contract printing are maturing, it is still unclear if 3D printing is cost-effective in all surgical oncology applications.

As of 2019, the Current Procedural Terminology (CPT) Editorial Board approved temporary (Category III) CPT codes for 3D printing. They are as follows: 0559T (for a model of one 3D-printed structure), 0560T (for each additional 3D-printed structure in the model), 0561T (for 3D-printed surgical guides), and 0562T (for each additional structure needed in the surgical guide).[25] These codes may be reimbursed by Medicare and potentially by private insurers.[25] After 5 years as temporary category III CPT codes, which are designated for emerging procedures, these codes are then eligible for conversion into category I CPT codes. However, such conversion requires significant longitudinal evidence, pending USFDA approval and must be considered common place.[25]

Given the novelty of 3D printing, large-scale data evaluating its effectiveness are still lacking. There are few studies based on randomized controlled designs and even fewer that compare long-term outcomes.[24] Thus, knowledge gaps remain as to the true impact that 3D-printed models may have on surgical practice.

Regulations on 3D-printed models in medicine are still in development. For example, the USFDA typically uses the 510(k) process to allow the use of 3D-printed models in surgery.[5] Three-dimensional-printed models are considered medical devices that are comparable to other iterations of similar models. Thus, 3D-printed models may undergo a less rigorous appraisal by the organization.[5] Some 3D-printed models for implantation are alternatively examined through the Humanitarian Use Device pathway.[5,26] This pathway is usually used by those deploying a device intended to treat a rare disease. With rare illnesses, robust and widespread testing of a particular device is often not possible. Thus, extensive efficacy data associated with specific 3D-printed models are still lacking.[26]

Finally, patient privacy is a potential issue. It is unclear if 3D reconstructions and 3D-printed models should be considered protected health information. This question has not been attended to by the Health Insurance Portability and Accountability Act.[27] Some aspects of 3D printing, particularly of internal structures, obviously are not easily reidentifiable but other anatomy, such as of the head and face, may be connected with a specific patient. Feldman and colleagues have recommended institutions develop their own privacy policies given the lack of more widespread regulatory policies.[27] Groups must decide how to best store and communicate information related to 3D reconstructions. Institutions must also protect any potentially patient identifiable information in 3D printing projects and use appropriate disposal methods when models are no longer needed.[27]

SUMMARY

The converging technologies of advanced medical imaging, computer-aided design, and 3D printing have enabled the rapid creations of patient-specific models that promise to further advance surgical oncology. Three-dimensional prints enhance patient and physician understandings of standard and diseased anatomy. Numerous applications of 3D prints have been explored in surgical oncology, ranging from preoperative planning to skills refinement, education, and creation of customized implants and surgical guides. Although there are measurable improvements associated with 3D-printed models such as improved patient understanding, decreased operative times, reduced radiation exposure, and decreased intraoperative blood loss, issues such as turnaround times, cost-effectiveness, materials availability, and long-term patient outcomes remain to be addressed. Much work remains for wider implementation of 3D printing in surgical oncology.

CLINICS CARE POINTS

1. Three-dimensional printing uses data from a patient's own imaging. Relevant structures from the imaging are segmented and then printed.

2. Three-dimensional printing can be a valuable resource for surgical planning in the setting of complex anatomy or unusual tumors.

3. Three-dimensional printing allows trainees and providers to practice and refine surgical skills through simulation.

4. Three-dimensional printing enables creation of durable tactile models incorporating biomimicry for improved understanding of basic and pathologic anatomy.

5. Three-dimensional printing can be used to create patient-specific surgical guides and implants.

6. Plan for leeway for turnaround time and learning curves when incorporating 3D printing into your educational endeavors or clinical practice.

7. Protect the privacy of the patient at all stages of developing and storing patient-specific models.

DISCLOSURE

The authors have nothing to disclose.

REFERENCES

1. Martelli N, Serrano C, van den Brink H, et al. Advantages and disadvantages of 3-dimensional printing in surgery: a systematic review. Surgery 2016;159(6): 1485–500.
2. Tejo-Otero A, Buj-Corral I, Fenollosa-Artés F. 3D printing in medicine for preoperative surgical planning: a review. Ann Biomed Eng 2020;48(2):536–55.
3. Mitsouras D, Liacouras P, Imanzadeh A, et al. Medical 3D printing for the radiologist. Radiographics 2015;35(7):1965–88.
4. Tack P, Victor J, Gemmel P, et al. 3D-printing techniques in a medical setting: a systematic literature review. Biomed Eng Online 2016;15:115.
5. Cheng GZ, San Jose Estepar R, Folch E, et al. Three-dimensional printing and 3D slicer. Chest 2016;149(5):1136–42.
6. Pugliese L, Marconi S, Negrello E, et al. The clinical use of 3D printing in surgery. Updates Surg 2018;70(3):381–8.
7. Ni J, Ling H, Zhang S, et al. Three-dimensional printing of metals for biomedical applications. Mater Today Bio 2019;3:100024.
8. Goldsmith I, Evans PL, Goodrum H, et al. Chest wall reconstruction with an anatomically designed 3-D printed titanium ribs and hemi-sternum implant. 3D Print Med 2020;6(1):26.
9. Pietrabissa A, Marconi S, Peri A, et al. From CT scanning to 3-D printing technology for the preoperative planning in laparoscopic splenectomy. Surg Endosc 2016;30(1):366–71.
10. Jones DB, Sung R, Weinberg C, et al. Three-dimensional modeling may improve surgical education and clinical practice. Surg Innov 2016;23(2):189–95.
11. Witowski JS, Pędziwiatr M, Major P, et al. Cost-effective, personalized, 3D-printed liver model for preoperative planning before laparoscopic liver hemihepatectomy for colorectal cancer metastases. Int J Comput Assist Radiol Surg 2017;12(12): 2047–54.
12. Garcia-Granero A, Sánchez-Guillén L, Fletcher-Sanfeliu D, et al. Application of three-dimensional printing in laparoscopic dissection to facilitate D3-lymphadenectomy for right colon cancer. Tech Coloproctol 2018;22(2):129–33.
13. Chen Y, Zhang J, Chen Q, et al. Three-dimensional printing technology for localised thoracoscopic segmental resection for lung cancer: a quasi-randomised clinical trial. World J Surg Oncol 2020;18(1):223.

14. Lui NS, Trope W, Guo HH, et al. 3D printed model of the mediastinum for cardio-thoracic surgery resident education. Presented at: Society of Thoracic Surgeons 57th Annual Meeting January 29, 2021; Virtual Meeting. 2021.

15. Marconi S, Pugliese L, Botti M, et al. Value of 3D printing for the comprehension of surgical anatomy. Surg Endosc 2017;31(10):4102–10.

16. Zheng YX, Yu DF, Zhao JG, Wu YL, et al. 3D printout models vs. 3D-rendered images: which is better for preoperative planning? J Surg Educ 2016;73(3):518–23.

17. Weinberg L, Pyo MH, Spanger M, et al. Personalised 3D-printed model of a chest-wall chondrosarcoma to enhance patient understanding of complex cardiothoracic surgery. BMJ Case Rep 2018;2018:bcr-2018–224464.

18. Yoon SH, Park S, Kang CH, et al. Personalized 3D-printed model for informed consent for stage i lung cancer: a randomized pilot trial. Semin Thorac Cardiovasc Surg 2019;31(2):316–8.

19. Sun W, Zhang L, Wang L, et al. Three-dimensionally printed template for percutaneous localization of multiple lung nodules. Ann Thorac Surg 2019;108(3):883–8.

20. Zhang L, Li M, Li Z, et al. Three-dimensional printing of navigational template in localization of pulmonary nodule: A pilot study. J Thorac Cardiovasc Surg 2017;154(6):2113–9.e7.

21. Zhang L, Wang L, Kadeer X, et al. Accuracy of a 3-dimensionally printed navigational template for localizing small pulmonary nodules. JAMA Surg 2019;154(4):295–303.

22. Dupret-Bories A, Vergez S, Meresse T, et al. Contribution of 3D printing to mandibular reconstruction after cancer. Eur Ann Otorhinolaryngol Head Neck Dis 2018;135(2):133–6.

23. Smelt J, Pontiki A, Jahangiri M, et al. Three-dimensional printing for chest wall reconstruction in thoracic surgery: building on experience. Thorac Cardiovasc Surg 2020;68(04):352–6.

24. Diment LE, Thompson MS, Bergmann JHM. Clinical efficacy and effectiveness of 3D printing: a systematic review. BMJ Open 2017;7(12):e016891.

25. Wake N. 3D printing for the radiologist, E-Book. Amsterdam: Elsevier Health Sciences; 2021.

26. Morrison RJ, Kashlan KN, Flanangan CL, et al. Regulatory considerations in the design and manufacturing of implantable 3D-printed medical devices. Clin Transl Sci 2015;8(5):594–600.

27. Feldman H, Kamali P, Lin SJ, et al. Clinical 3D printing: a protected health information (PHI) and compliance perspective. Int J Med Inf 2018;115:18–23.

Intraoperative Molecular Imaging of Lung Cancer
A Review

Natalie S. Lui, MD[a],*, Sunil Singhal, MD[b]

KEYWORDS

- Intraoperative molecular imaging • Fluorescence imaging • Thoracic surgery
- Indocyanine green • OTL38 • Panitumumab-IRDye800

KEY POINTS

- Intraoperative molecular imaging is a promising technology in the surgical treatment of lung cancer. It involves a cancer-targeted fluorescent imaging contrast agent that accumulates in the tumor and a camera that detects that imaging agent.
- Imaging agents are either receptor-targeted or nonreceptor-targeted, and they fluoresce in the near-infrared or visible light spectrum. The most promising agents are very specific to the tumor and fluoresce in the near-infrared spectrum, leading to a higher tumor-to-background ratio.
- OTL38 is an imaging agent that targets the folate receptor, which is overexpressed in lung adenocarcinoma and fluoresces in the near-infrared spectrum.
- An initial clinical trial of OTL38 showed promising results, with a 24% rate of a clinically significant event such as the identification of the primary tumor, additional tumor, or positive margin that was not otherwise found using traditional methods.

INTRODUCTION

Lung cancer is the most common cause of cancer-related death in the United States, and surgical resection is the mainstay of the treatment of early-stage disease. The 5-year overall survival ranges from 92% for patients with stage IA1 disease to less than 10% for patients with stage IV disease.[1] Most cases of early-stage disease are first identified on computed tomography (CT) scans obtained for unrelated reasons[2] or low-dose screening CT scans performed in high-risk patients.[3,4] When a nodule is

[a] Department of Cardiothoracic Surgery, Stanford University School of Medicine, 300 Pasteur Drive, Falk Building, Stanford, CA 94305, USA; [b] Division of Thoracic Surgery, Translational Research, Department of Surgery, University of Pennsylvania, 3400 Civic Center Boulevard, 14th Floor, PCAM South Tower, Philadelphia, PA, USA
* Corresponding author.
E-mail address: natalielui@stanford.edu
Twitter: @natalielui22 (N.S.L.)

Surg Oncol Clin N Am 31 (2022) 685–693
https://doi.org/10.1016/j.soc.2022.06.006
1055-3207/22/© 2022 Elsevier Inc. All rights reserved.

found, percutaneous CT-guided or bronchoscopic biopsy is often performed to confirm a cancer diagnosis. If this biopsy is nondiagnostic, or if the lung nodule is suspicious enough to forego the less invasive biopsy, a surgical biopsy is performed. This procedure is usually a sublobar resection (either wedge resection or segmentectomy) performed with a minimally invasive approach (either video-assisted thoracoscopic surgery [VATS] or robot-assisted thoracoscopic surgery). For early-stage disease in the periphery of the lung, sublobar resection is not only diagnostic but also therapeutic. For more advanced tumors, once the surgical biopsy confirms cancer, a completion lobectomy is performed.

During sublobar resections, surgeons must identify the suspicious lung nodule to remove the correct part of the lung with adequate margins. However, localization is difficult when the nodules are small, part solid, or far from the pleural surface. Landmarks are difficult to use during surgery because the lung is collapsed on the side of surgery during the operation. In addition, it is more difficult to palpate the lung during minimally invasive surgery compared with traditional open surgery performed through a larger incision (thoracotomy).

Many methods of preoperative localization of lung nodules have been developed but they all have disadvantages. Most commonly, patients undergo CT-guided placement of a hookwire[5] or fiducial marker or injection of methylene blue dye or a radiotracer.[6] These procedures are performed in a radiology suite and must be coordinated with the operating rooms. They expose the patient to radiation, as well as the risk of pneumothorax or lung hemorrhage. Afterward, the wire could be dislodged, or the dye could spread beyond the tumor, making the procedure less useful. The fiducial requires fluoroscopic guidance during surgery, and the radiotracer requires a surgical gamma probe, both of which can be cumbersome to use. Another option is injection of dye under bronchoscopic guidance, usually using electromagnetic navigation systems that require specialized mapping of the operating room.[7,8] Clearly, we need better methods for intraoperative localization of lung nodules.

Intraoperative molecular imaging (IMI) is a promising technique for tumor identification and other applications. The method relies on an imaging agent, which is usually given systemically and accumulates within the tumor, as well as a fluorescence camera that detects the signal from that agent during surgery. The imaging agents are typically targeted to the tumor and not based on vascular perfusion that has been used historically. Targeting of the fluorochromes to the tumor can either be based on specific receptors or on more global properties of the tumor that are not receptor specific. Receptor-targeted agents are composed of a probe (which targets the specific molecule of interest in the tumor) conjugated to a dye (which fluoresces at a certain wavelength). The probes are molecules of various sizes, from small peptides to larger antibodies. The signal detected by the camera is represented as a tumor-to-background ratio (TBR), calculated by dividing the mean fluorescence intensity (MFI) of the tumor by the MFI of the adjacent normal tissue. Various imaging agents and cameras have been tested in different types of cancer, with the goals of tumor localization, confirmation of negative margins, identification of positive lymph nodes, and discovery of additional disease not seen on traditional preoperative imaging. In thoracic surgery, several imaging agents have been studied but they are still in the research setting. OTL38, which targets the folate receptor and uses a near-infrared fluorophore, is currently undergoing an ongoing randomized trial. In addition, there is a carcinoembryonic antigen (CEA)-receptor-specific targeted fluorochromes that is in a pilot study for CEA + lung cancers.

We will review data on IMI of lung cancer. Four imaging agents have been studied in clinical trials enrolling patients with lung cancer[1]: indocyanine green (ICG), which is nontargeted and near-infrared[2]; EC17, which is targeted and not near-infrared[3]; OTL38, which is targeted and near-infrared; and[4] panitumumab-IRDye800. The results have shown great promise for the surgical treatment of lung cancer, as well as several limitations of the technology.

INDOCYANINE GREEN

In lung cancer, the first-studied IMI agent was ICG, a nonreceptor-targeted, near-infrared agent with excitation wavelength of 805 nm and emission wavelength of 830 nm.[9] It was approved by the Food and Drug Administration (FDA) in 1959 and remains the only approved near-infrared agent. Most near-infrared surgical cameras were developed for ICG imaging. Because ICG is nontargeted and not tumor specific, most applications assess tissue perfusion alone using ICG at a low dose (5–10 mg) administered by intravenous push followed by a saline flush minutes before imaging.[10,11] Within thoracic surgery, for example, it has been used to determine the intersegmental plane during segmentectomy and to evaluate for gastric conduit ischemia during esophagectomy. ICG has also been injected directly into the tumor using CT[12] or bronchoscopic guidance[13] for intraoperative tumor localization.

In contrast, for IMI of lung cancer, ICG has been given at a much higher dose (5 mg/kg) via infusion 24 hours before surgery (named "TumorGlow" to differentiate it from the lower dose for measuring perfusion). The accumulation of ICG within tumors is thought to rely on the enhanced permeability and retention effect more than tissue perfusion. This phenomenon describes passive accumulation of macromolecules (in this case, ICG bound to albumin) in tumors after they extravasate from leaky capillaries.[14–16]

Okusanya and colleagues[17] conducted a trial of 18 patients undergoing surgical resection of lung cancer who received an ICG infusion 5 mg/kg at 24 hours before surgery (**Fig. 1**). All operations were performed via a thoracotomy incision, and the fluorescence camera system was constructed in the laboratory for the trial.[18] IMI detected 14 out of 18 known nodules of a wide variety of histologies and even identified 5 additional nodules that were not seen on preoperative imaging, with the mean TBR 2.2 (range, 1.5–4.4). However, the depth of penetration was shown to be a potential limitation of the technology; the deepest nodule with fluorescence was 1.3 cm from the pleural surface; and of the 4 nodules that were not identified intraoperatively, 2 had ex vivo fluorescence when the lung was incised. Another major problem with this approach was highly anthracotic lungs in heavy smokers had significant noise from background inflammation in the lung.

Holt and colleagues[19] also conducted a trial of 5 patients scheduled for lung resection for cancer in which they gave ICG preoperatively and examined the specimens

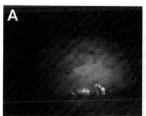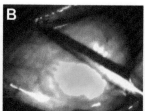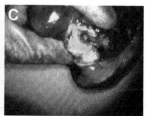

Fig. 1. Example of indocyanine green (ICG) targeting of a lung nodule. (*A*) View of the lung nodule with (*A*) white and (*B*) near-infrared light. (*C*) Backtable examination of the lung nodule with near-infrared light after bisection.

ex vivo. All tumors had good fluorescence signaling with the mean signal-to-background ratio (SBR) 8.1, and the fluorescence was homogeneous throughout the tumor. However, the one tumor that had peritumoral atelectasis showed that the fluorescence signal was also present in the surrounding inflammation (SBR 5.6 compared with SBR 8.9 of the tumor). This study demonstrated a potential limitation of using a nontargeted agent, which ICG accumulated in peritumoral inflammation.

Mao and colleagues[20] later confirmed the potential of IMI of lung cancer using ICG. They enrolled 36 patients with non-small cell lung cancer or metastatic lung cancer scheduled for lung resection of at least one lung nodule and used the same regimen, 5 mg/kg via infusion 24 hours before surgery. In this trial, the patients underwent VATS approaches, and the 2 fluorescence camera systems D-light P system (Karl Storz, Goleta, CA), SUPEREYE system (Key Laboratory of Molecular Imaging, Chinese Academy of Science) were designed for minimally invasive surgery, one commercial and one developed in their laboratory. IMI was able to detect 68 of 76 nodules in vivo, including 9 nodules that were not detected by white light exploration. Promisingly, nodules as small as 1 mm were detected, and the SBR was high even for nodules 1 cm or smaller (3.14 ± 1.59). However, the depth of penetration continued to be a concern because they could not detect 8 nodules that were 1.3 cm or more from the pleural surface. Of note, the SBR was higher in lung squamous cell carcinoma than adenocarcinoma (4.08 vs 2.91).

Kim and colleagues[21] conducted a smaller trial of 11 patients scheduled for VATS lung resection of primary or metastatic lung cancer using a smaller dose of ICG 1 mg/kg given intravenously 24 hours before surgery. They did not perform IMI but imaged specimens using a commercially available camera on the backtable. Fluorescence signal was detected in 10 of 11 specimens with MFI 5.1 ± 3.3, including a 2.2 cm adenocarcinoma located 14 mm deep. The only nodule without fluorescence signal was a 2.9 cm squamous cell carcinoma and located 12 mm deep. Among the 10 nodules with fluorescence, the MFI was not correlated with tumor size or maximum standardized uptake value (SUV_{max}). Another potential limitation was demonstrated: 2 specimens without residual tumor showed high fluorescence signals in areas of obstructive pneumonia with MFI 8.2 and 9, respectively.

These findings demonstrated that ICG had good fluorescence signaling in lung cancer but had several important limitations. Fluorescence signaling in peritumoral inflammation highlighted the need for a targeted imaging agent and the limited depth of penetration the need for a near-infrared agent.

EC17

As a nonreceptor-targeted imaging agent, ICG was found to accumulate in peritumoral inflammation, potentially a major limitation in IMI. Thus, targeted imaging agents were thought to be more promising in clinical applications. Two imaging agents studied next were folate analogs that targeted the folate receptor, which is highly expressed in certain cancers including lung adenocarcinomas.[22,23] EC17 (On Target Laboratories, West Lafayette, IN) is a folate analog conjugated to fluorescein isothiocyanate, a fluorophore in the visible light spectrum with an excitation wavelength of 470 nm and emission wavelength of 520 nm.[24]

Kennedy and colleagues[25] performed a study of 30 patients given an EC17 infusion 0.1 mg/kg 4 hours before diagnostic wedge resection for indeterminant lung nodules. Ex vivo IMI showed fluorescence in all 19 nodules determined to be adenocarcinoma on final pathologic condition and no fluorescence in the remaining 11 nodules. In fact, this so-called optical biopsy was more accurate than frozen section analysis, which only identified 13 of the 19 as adenocarcinoma, and 5 of the remaining 6 as malignant. One patient had fluorescence on molecular imaging but no evidence of malignancy on frozen section, and permanent section confirmed adenocarcinoma; they subsequently returned to the operating room for completion lobectomy. In addition to being more accurate, the optical biopsy was faster as well, taking an average time of 2.4 minutes compared with 26.5 minutes for frozen section.

Okusanya et al[26] then performed a study of 50 patients given an EC17 infusion 0.1 mg/kg 4 hours before open surgery for lung adenocarcinoma. In vivo IMI identified only 7 tumors intraoperatively, with the mean TBR 3.6 ± 1.2. Of the remaining 43 tumors, 39 had ex vivo fluorescence, with the mean TBR 4.2 ± 2.7. In addition, TBR of tumors near the pleural surface (<1.2 cm) was greater than that of tumors deeper in the lung ($P = .044$). On pathologic analysis, the 46 tumors that had in situ or ex vivo fluorescence all expressed the folate receptor, and the 4 tumors that were not fluorescent did not express the folate receptor.

These findings demonstrated that EC17 was indeed localizing to lung adenocarcinomas that expressed the folate receptor but a fluorophore in the visible light spectrum has poor tissue penetration. In addition, there was significant autofluorescence in the chest, mainly from the bronchus and pulmonary artery.[27] Due to this major limitation of a visible wavelength fluorochromes, the agent was abandoned. These results showed that a near-infrared imaging agent would be better for imaging nodules in the lung.

OTL38

After the less promising results with ICG, which was near-infrared but not receptor-targeted, and EC17, which was targeted but not near-infrared, a new imaging agent that was both targeted and near-infrared was developed. This agent, known as OTL38 (On Target Laboratories, West Lafayette, IN), is another folate analog conjugated to S0456, a fluorophore in the near-infrared spectrum with an excitation wavelength of 774 to 776 nm and emission wavelength of 794 to 796 nm.[28] The near-infrared dyes have several advantages. They provide greater TBR because light in the visible range (400–700 nm) is absorbed by hemoglobin and light greater than 900 nm is absorbed by water or lipids. In addition, they do not generate as much autofluorescence.[29] They also have deeper tissue penetration depth than the dyes with wavelengths in the visible range, which is critical for tumors deep in the lung.[30] Finally, near-infrared imaging is especially suited to minimally invasive surgery: the surgeon is already using a monitor, there is little ambient light, and the fluorescence imaging system can be built into the surgical cameras.[29]

Gangadharan and colleagues[31] performed a multicenter phase II trial of 92 patients undergoing surgery for lung adenocarcinoma (**Fig. 2**). OTL38 infusion 0.025 mg/kg was given 2 to 6 hours before surgery. Clinically significant events were defined as

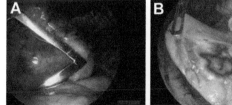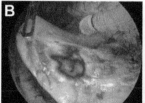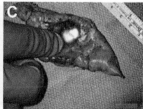

Fig. 2. Example of an OTL38 targeting of a lung nodule. (*A*) View of the lung nodule with (*A*) white light and (*B*) near-infrared light. (*C*) Backtable examination of the lung nodule with near-infrared light.

a change in the operation due to IMI: identification of the primary nodule when it could not be found with the usual white light inspection and palpation, identification of an additional nodule that is malignant, or identification of a true-positive margin. IMI led to at least one predefined clinically significant event in 24 (26%) patients. There were 13 cases in which the surgeon could not identify the lung nodule by visualization or palpation, and 11 of these were found with molecular imaging. There were 9 additional cancers found, which changed the stage in 7 patients. There were 16 cases with fluorescence within 5 mm of the margin, and 9 of these had a positive margin on pathologic review.

The study was the first multicenter trial of IMI of lung cancer, and the results clearly show the benefits of IMI over our traditional surgical techniques. They also demonstrated that surgeons could adopt this technology quickly; all surgeons were comfortable with IMI by 10 cases, and the average time used for IMI was 15 minutes.

The potential limitations of OTL38 included the limited depth of penetration (estimated 2–3 cm), a false-positive signal in the lymph node and near the lung hilum, and a 20% rate of adverse events during infusion. In addition, OTL38 is expected to be useful only in adenocarcinoma; whereas 74% of lung adenocarcinomas were shown to express the folate receptor, only 13% of lung squamous cell carcinomas had any folate receptor expression in at least 5% of the tumor.[22]

A randomized trial of OTL38 (NCT04241315) was recently completed and we are awaiting results. All patients received OTL38 injection and then were randomized to undergo intraoperative imaging or not. The primary endpoint was again a clinically significant event, defined as an intraoperative finding during surgery that altered the course of the operation.

PANITUMUMAB-IRDye800

Another imaging agent being studied in lung cancer is panitumumab-IRDye800. It is a conjugate of the epidermal growth factor receptor (EGFR) antibody panitumumab and the near-infrared dye IRDye800.[32] Fakurnejad et al[33] and van Keulen et al[34] studied panitumumab-IRDye800 in patients with head and neck cancer to predict margin and lymph node status.[35] They found that 56% of head and neck squamous cell carcinoma specimens have a moderate-to-intense EGFR expression in the tumor.[36]

Panitumumab is a promising probe for lung cancer because EGFR is a transmembrane tyrosine kinase that regulates cell growth and is frequently overexpressed in lung cancer.[37,38] It is expected to accumulate even in lung cancers with EGFR mutations because those mutations occur in the intracellular domain.[39] In addition, antibody-based imaging agents have several advantage.[40] FDA-approved antibodies have well-known pharmacokinetic and toxicity profiles; because the required dose for imaging is often less than for treatment, the adverse events associated with antibody-based imaging agents are expected to be far fewer than with the antibodies alone. In fact, the half-life (days to weeks) is much longer than that of the smaller imaging agents, allowing more specific targeting of cancer cells. Finally, they can be labeled with various fluorescent probes and could potentially be used in combinations.

SUMMARY

Molecular imaging is a developing field in surgical oncology with the potential to change the surgical treatment of lung cancer. Potential applications of IMI include tumor localization, confirmation of negative margins, identification of positive lymph nodes, and discovery of additional disease not seen on traditional preoperative imaging. These techniques will be even more important as thoracic surgeons are performing more minimally invasive operations, which do not allow thorough palpation compared with open approaches, and more sublobar resections, in which margin status is key. They also have several advantages such as no radiation exposure to the patient or health-care team and the ability to use standard endoscopes for fluorescence imaging. Development of IMI in lung cancer will require understanding of its limitations, such as depth of penetration and false-positive fluorescence from peritumoral inflammation, hilar structures, and autofluorescence.

The future of this field will likely involve more targeted dyes to visualize squamous cell carcinomas and other histologies. Moreover, cameras with lasers that can get deeper lung penetration are rapidly coming into the space. Finally, alterations to the fluorochromes in the contrast agents will allow deeper penetration. One of the major challenges that has not been solved is identifying the micrometastatic disease in the lymph nodes.

CLINICS CARE POINTS

- Intraoperative molecular imaging will be particularly helpful as thoracic surgeons perform more minimally invasive, sublobar resections for lung cancer.

- Standard endoscopes and robotic cameras now allow surgeons to switch quickly between white light and fluorescence modes.

- There are currently no approved imaging agents for lung cancer. OTL38 is a targeted, near-infrared agent in phase III clinical trials.

DISCLOSURE

N.S. Lui has a research grant from the Intuitive Foundation, United States. S. Singhal has no disclosures.

REFERENCES

1. Detterbeck FC, Boffa DJ, Kim AW, et al. The eighth edition lung cancer stage classification. Chest 2017;151(1):193–203.
2. Seidelman JL, Myers JL, Quint LE. Incidental, subsolid pulmonary nodules at CT: etiology and management. Cancer Imaging 2013;13(3):365–73.
3. The National Lung Screening Trial Research Team. Reduced lung-cancer mortality with low-dose computed tomographic screening. N Engl J Med 2011;365(5): 395–409.
4. de Koning HJ, van der Aalst CM, de Jong PA, et al. Reduced lung-cancer mortality with volume CT screening in a randomized trial. N Engl J Med 2020; 382(6):503–13.
5. Zhao G, Yu X, Chen W, et al. Computed tomography-guided preoperative semi-rigid hook-wire localization of small pulmonary nodules: 74 cases report. J Cardiothorac Surg 2019;14:149. Available at: https://www.ncbi.nlm.nih.gov/pmc/articles/PMC6701050/.
6. Burdine J, Joyce LD, Plunkett MB, et al. Feasibility and value of video-assisted thoracoscopic surgery wedge excision of small pulmonary nodules in patients with malignancy. Chest 2002;122(4):1467–70.
7. Marino KA, Sullivan JL, Weksler B. Electromagnetic navigation bronchoscopy for identifying lung nodules for thoracoscopic resection. Ann Thorac Surg 2016; 102(2):454–7.

8. Abbas A, Kadakia S, Ambur V, et al. Intraoperative electromagnetic navigational bronchoscopic localization of small, deep, or subsolid pulmonary nodules. J Thorac Cardiovasc Surg 2017;153(6):1581–90.

9. Okusanya OT, Hess NR, Luketich JD, et al. Infrared intraoperative fluorescence imaging using indocyanine green in thoracic surgery. Eur J Cardiothorac Surg 2018;53(3):512–8.

10. Chiu C-H, Chao Y-K, Liu Y-H, et al. Clinical use of near-infrared fluorescence imaging with indocyanine green in thoracic surgery: a literature review. J Thorac Dis 2016;8(Suppl 9):S744–8.

11. Pardolesi A, Veronesi G, Solli P, et al. Use of indocyanine green to facilitate intersegmental plane identification during robotic anatomic segmentectomy. J Thorac Cardiovasc Surg 2014;148(2):737–8.

12. Wu Z, Zhang L, Zhao X, et al. Localization of subcentimeter pulmonary nodules using an indocyanine green near-infrared imaging system during uniportal video-assisted thoracoscopic surgery. J Cardiothorac Surg 2021;16:224.

13. Hachey KJ, Digesu CS, Armstrong KW, et al. A novel technique for tumor localization and targeted lymphatic mapping in early-stage lung cancer. J Thorac Cardiovasc Surg 2017;154(3):1110–8.

14. Matsumura Y, Maeda H. A New Concept for Macromolecular Therapeutics in Cancer Chemotherapy: Mechanism of Tumoritropic Accumulation of Proteins and the Antitumor Agent Smancs. Cancer Research 1986;46:6387–92.

15. Maeda H, Matsumura Y. EPR effect based drug design and clinical outlook for enhanced cancer chemotherapy. Adv Drug Deliv Rev 2011;63(3):129–30.

16. Heneweer C, Holland JP, Divilov V, et al. Magnitude of enhanced permeability and retention effect in tumors with different phenotypes: [89] Zr-Albumin as a model SYSTEM. J Nucl Med 2011;52(4):625–33.

17. Okusanya OT, Holt D, Heitjan D, et al. Intraoperative near-infrared imaging can identify pulmonary nodules. Ann Thorac Surg 2014;98(4):1223–30.

18. Okusanya OT, Madajewski B, Segal E, et al. Small portable interchangeable imager of fluorescence for fluorescence guided surgery and research. Technol Cancer Res Treat 2015;14(2):213–20.

19. Holt D, Okusanya O, Judy R, et al. Intraoperative near-infrared imaging can distinguish cancer from normal tissue but not inflammation. Multhoff G, editor. PLoS One 2014;9(7):e103342.

20. Mao Y, Chi C, Yang F, et al. The identification of sub-centimetre nodules by near-infrared fluorescence thoracoscopic systems in pulmonary resection surgeries. Eur J Cardiothorac Surg 2017;52(6):1190–6.

21. Kim HK, Quan YH, Choi BH, et al. Intraoperative pulmonary neoplasm identification using near-infrared fluorescence imaging. Eur J Cardiothorac Surg 2016; 49(5):1497–502.

22. O'Shannessy DJ, Yu G, Smale R, et al. Folate receptor alpha expression in lung cancer: diagnostic and prognostic significance. Oncotarget 2012;3(4):414–25.

23. Elnakat H. Distribution, functionality and gene regulation of folate receptor isoforms: implications in targeted therapy. Adv Drug Deliv Rev 2004;56(8):1067–84.

24. De Jesus E, Keating JJ, Kularatne SA, et al. Comparison of folate receptor targeted optical contrast agents for intraoperative molecular imaging. Int J Mol Imaging 2015;2015:1–10.

25. Kennedy GT, Okusanya OT, Keating JJ, et al. The optical biopsy: a novel technique for rapid intraoperative diagnosis of primary pulmonary adenocarcinomas. Ann Surg 2015;262(4):602–9.

26. Okusanya OT, DeJesus EM, Jiang JX, et al. Intraoperative molecular imaging can identify lung adenocarcinomas during pulmonary resection. J Thorac Cardiovasc Surg 2015;150(1):28–35.e1.

27. Predina JD, Okusanya O, D Newton A, et al. Standardization and optimization of intraoperative molecular imaging for identifying primary pulmonary adenocarcinomas. Mol Imaging Biol 2018;20(1):131–8.

28. Predina JD, Newton AD, Keating J, et al. A phase I clinical trial of targeted intraoperative molecular imaging for pulmonary adenocarcinomas. Ann Thorac Surg 2018;105(3):901–8.

29. Rosenthal EL, Warram JM, Bland KI, et al. The status of contemporary image-guided modalities in oncologic surgery. Ann Surg 2015;261(1):46–55.

30. Adams KE, Ke S, Kwon S, et al. Comparison of visible and near-infrared wavelength-excitable fluorescent dyes for molecular imaging of cancer. J Biomed Opt 2007;12(2):024017.

31. Gangadharan S, Sarkaria I, Rice D, et al. Multi-institutional Phase 2 clinical trial of intraoperative molecular imaging of lung cancer. Ann Thorac Surg 2021;112(4): 1150–9. S0003497520319317.

32. Bhattacharyya S, Patel N, Wei L, et al. Synthesis and biological evaluation of panitumumab-IRDye800 conjugate as a fluorescence imaging probe for EGFR-expressing cancers. MedChemComm 2014;5(9):1337–46.

33. Fakurnejad S, Krishnan G, van Keulen S, et al. Intraoperative molecular imaging for ex vivo assessment of peripheral margins in oral squamous cell carcinoma. Front Oncol 2019;9:1476.

34. van Keulen S, van den Berg NS, Nishio N, et al. Rapid, non-invasive fluorescence margin assessment: Optical specimen mapping in oral squamous cell carcinoma. Oral Oncol 2019;88:58–65.

35. Nishio N, van den Berg NS, van Keulen S, et al. Optical molecular imaging can differentiate metastatic from benign lymph nodes in head and neck cancer. Nat Commun 2019;10(1):5044.

36. Sweeny L, Dean NR, Magnuson JS, et al. EGFR expression in advanced head and neck cutaneous squamous cell carcinoma. Head Neck 2012;34(5):681–6.

37. Bethune G, Bethune D, Ridgway N, et al. Epidermal growth factor receptor (EGFR) in lung cancer: an overview and update. J Thorac Dis 2010;2(1):48–51.

38. Nakamura H. Survival impact of epidermal growth factor receptor overexpression in patients with non-small cell lung cancer: a meta-analysis. Thorax 2006;61(2): 140–5.

39. Herbst RS, Heymach JV, Lippman SM. Lung cancer. N Engl J Med 2008;359: 1367–80.

40. Warram JM, de Boer E, Sorace AG, et al. Antibody-based imaging strategies for cancer. Cancer Metastasis Rev 2014;33(2–3):809–22.

Current and Future Applications of Fluorescence-Guided Surgery in Head and Neck Cancer

Estelle Martin, Marisa Hom, PhD, Lucas Mani, MS,
Eben L. Rosenthal, MD*

KEYWORDS

- Fluorescence-guided surgery • Near-infrared imaging • Nonspecific fluorophores
- Tumor-targeting fluorophores • Positive surgical margins

KEY POINTS

- Positive surgical margins remain at 30% in head and neck cancer resections and are associated with a 90% increase in local occurrence and, in some head and neck cancers, a significant increase in 5-year mortality rate.
- In the past decade, surgical oncologists have turned to molecular imaging in fluorescence-guided surgery—a technique for enhanced intraoperative tumor identification.
- The emergence of tumor-targeting fluorophores foreshadows exciting progress for intraoperative imaging during head and neck cancer resections.

INTRODUCTION

The treatment of head and neck cancer (HNC)—the sixth most common cancer worldwide—requires a multidisciplinary approach.[1] Standard of care in advanced HNC typically includes surgical resection of solid tumors and subsequent adjuvant radiotherapy or chemoradiotherapy.[2] Treatment success largely hinges on complete resection of malignant tissue during surgery. Positive surgical margins are associated with a 90% increase in local occurrence and, in some HNCs, a significant increase in 5-year mortality rate.[3,4] Given that surgeons depend on subtle visual cues, palpation, and frozen section analysis (FSA) to determine the status of surgical margins, it is not surprising that these techniques have yielded positive margins in up to 30% of all HNC resections. Despite improvements in medical management of these cancers, positive

Department of Otolaryngology–Head and Neck Surgery, Vanderbilt University Medical Center, Preston Research Building 754, 2220 Pierce Avenue, Nashville, TN 37232, USA
* Corresponding author. 1215 21st Avenue South, Suite 6310, Nashville, TN 37232.
E-mail address: e.rosenthal@vumc.org

Surg Oncol Clin N Am 31 (2022) 695–706
https://doi.org/10.1016/j.soc.2022.07.001
1055-3207/22/© 2022 Elsevier Inc. All rights reserved.

surgonc.theclinics.com

margin rates have remained relatively unchanged in the past 30 years, emphasizing a need for improved intraoperative imaging and tumor visualization for HNCs.[5] Until recently, visualization of malignant disease was limited to anatomical imaging systems such as PET, computed tomography (CT), MRI, and ultrasonography—all of which are predominantly performed in the context of preoperative planning. In the past decade, surgical oncologists have turned to molecular imaging in fluorescence-guided surgery (FGS)—a technique for enhanced intraoperative tumor identification (**Fig. 1**).[6] This review evaluates the development of tumor-specific fluorophores that have emerged onto the FGS field including the evolving landscape, current methods, and future potential of FGS in the head and neck oncological field.[7]

CONVENTIONAL IMAGING METHODS

Anatomic imaging modalities such as CT and MRI have been standard in preoperative evaluation in oncological imaging for several decades.[8] MRI is shown to display comparatively better soft tissue contrast than CT; however, it is limited by its lengthy scan time and dependence on patient immobility.[9] Iodinated intravenous contrast media can be used to enhance CT images, whereas gadolinium-based contrast materials can be used for MRI—both of which illuminate the patient's vascular pathways.[8] Intraoperative use of CT and MRI has been widely used by orthopedic services and glioblastoma services, respectively. However, contrast enhancement is logistically and technically challenging in the intraoperative setting as described in later discussion.

The value of tumor-specific imaging methods for tumor visualization and oncological treatment has been established by PET. First performed in 1976, it eventually became a primary nuclear imaging modality for the identification of malignant cancers.[10–12] 18F-fluorodeoxyglucose (^{18}F-FDG) is currently the most common radiotracer used for tumor-detecting PET scans.[13] The high glycolytic rate of cancer cells remains fundamental to the success of tumor detection in PET scans; ^{18}F-FDG PET scans detect abnormally high absorption of radiotracer in cancer cells, due to their heightened metabolic rates and sugar consumption.[11] Compared with PET, CT

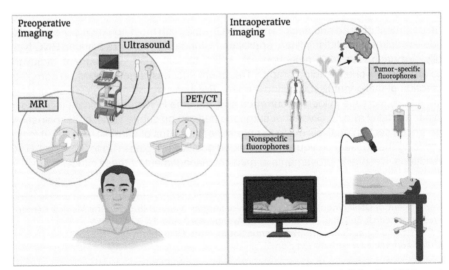

Fig. 1. Utilization of preoperative and intraoperative imaging modalities for HNC treatment. (Image created using BioRender.)

and MRI offer higher-resolution anatomic imaging of solid tumors and a spatial map of the surrounding structures, but fail to provide the sensitivity to detect tumor, especially in patients with posttreatment anatomic distortions, which is the value of PET.[12,14]

Ultrasonography is an additional tool for oncological imaging. This system was originally developed for obstetric and gynecologic purposes in 1958; however, the machine's ability to capture soft tissue disease has made it a valuable tool for visualizing and diagnosing malignancies.[15–17]

Intraoperative Hurdles

In the past 2 decades, the standard of care for evaluation and surveillance of regional and metastatic disease in HNC has combined CT and PET imaging modalities—[18]FDG-PET/CT—for a more exhaustive representation of disease progression.[12] The combination of these 2 imaging systems allows oncologists to bridge the gap between anatomic and physiologic visualization of malignant disease. These scans are highly sensitive but lack specificity (sensitivity—T: 97%–100%, N: 82%–87%, M: 53%–100%; specificity—T: 94%, N: 79%–86%, M: 93%–98%). Interrogation of false-positive lesions leads to unnecessary procedures, overdiagnosis/upstaging, patient anxiety, increased cost, and repeat imaging.

Furthermore, although PET, CT, MRI, and ultrasonography are crucial evaluative tools for preoperative staging, using these imaging modalities in the operating theater poses significant challenges. Despite its capacity to capture high-resolution scans in full-body imaging, CT imaging cannot be used in real time and does not image soft tissue or solid tumors without contrast, which is technically difficult to administer in the operating room. Furthermore, resolution of CT bone imaging is comparatively inferior to human vision (50 μm).[18] Real-time detection of radionuclides using handheld PET detector imaging has very poor resolution on the order of centimeters. Although ultrasound resolution (<30 μm) overcomes this concern, the instrument's necessary tissue contact, nonspecific contrast, dependence on user experience, and relatively small field of view pose additional challenges in the operating room.[18] Finally, most of these imaging systems—MRI, CT, and PET especially—are very large and require specialized operating suites to accommodate their size.[19] These various shortcomings emphasize the demand for intraoperative imaging tools with better specificity and ease of use.

MOLECULAR IMAGING METHODS
Nonspecific Optical Agents

Intraoperative optical imaging has been rapidly developed within surgical oncology within the last 20 years with 4 US Food and Drug Administration (FDA)-approved nonspecific optical agents, a recent tumor-targeting optical agent, and more than a dozen agents in phase 2 or later clinical trials.

Fluorescence imaging is complementary to preoperative imaging modalities. Although PET, CT, and/or MRI can be used to plan surgical approach and determine resectability, intraoperative fluorescent agents illuminate the tumor, providing direct visualization of small fragments of tumor in real-time intraoperative feedback, including positive tumor margins.[18] When fluorescent contrast optical agents are administered to the patient, an exogenous fluorescence excitation light source is required to trigger molecules to absorb photons.[20] This excitation prompts the subsequent emission of photons at a longer wavelength, producing a fluorescent signal that is ultimately captured by a detector array (**Fig. 2**).[18,21] Imaging in the near-infrared (NIR) (700–1000 nm) spectrum has proved particularly advantageous in FGS due to

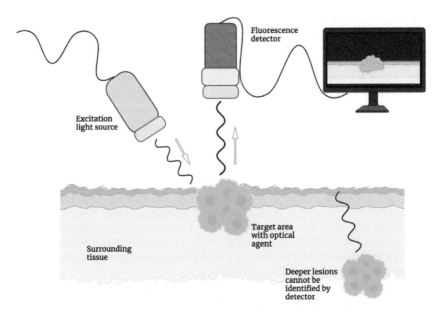

Fig. 2. Basic FGS optical mechanism. (Image created using BioRender.)

high tissue penetration (up to 2 cm) and low autofluorescence in background tissues.[18,21,22]

FDA-approved nonspecific fluorophores used for general cancer imaging include indocyanine green (ICG), 5- aminolevulinic acid (5-ALA), methylene blue, and fluorescein isothiocyanate (FITC).[21] At present, only ICG is approved and routinely used for intravenous administration. As a hydrophobic agent, it immediately binds to plasma proteins, confining the molecule to the vascular compartment, which makes it a commonly used intraoperative measure of vascular perfusion in plastic surgery.[22] Because ICG is nonspecific, its success as a cancer imaging agent depends on leaky vasculature characteristic of many solid tumors.[21,23] As a result, ICG tends to accumulate in tumor regions—a phenomenon known as the enhanced permeability and retention effect—providing surgeons with real-time feedback on the surgical field.[23] ICG is currently the most widely used fluorophore in surgical applications.[24]

Methylene blue is an additional nonspecific contrast dye with a peak emission wavelength just below the NIR range (688 nm), thus it can be seen by the naked eye.[25] Although not systemically injected for imaging purposes, it is directly injected into the tumor and typically paired with radioisotope for sentinel lymph node (SLN) mapping among patients with melanoma and breast cancer.[21,23,26] It must be noted that the use of ICG and methylene blue for evaluation of the SLN requires intratumoral dye injection and subsequent observation of the drainage pattern—a procedure that reduces operative flow and is often painful for the patient.[10,27]

5-ALA is an amino acid that is currently approved for use in FGS for high-grade gliomas and works by capitalizing on the high metabolic activity of cancer cells.[21,28] After oral administration, 5-ALA is rapidly processed by the heme synthesis pathway in tumor tissues, and thus produces elevated concentrations of protoporphyrin IX—a molecule with an emission peak (635 nm) in the red visible light range—in these regions.[21,23] Hexaminolevulinate, the hexyl ester of 5-ALA, exhibits similar mechanisms. This imaging agent has been approved for topical application within the bladder for visualization of bladder cancer.[29] Finally, FITC is a fluorescein derivative with a peak absorbance value similar to that of hemoglobin (521 nm); however, the fluorophore itself is not used alone for tumor imaging.[27,30]

Although these agents have been used for FGS, they are limited by their nontargeted nature; that is, the agents themselves are not cancer selective.[23] In addition, 5-ALA, FITC, and methylene blue fluorophores emit photons outside of the NIR range, resulting in decreased penetration depth and higher autofluorescence from nontumor tissue, and as suboptimal intraoperative imaging agents have not been widely adopted. To address these issues, research efforts have turned to fluorophore-conjugated molecular probes with a high affinity to unique cancer targets for enhanced differentiation between normal and cancerous tissue.[14,18]

Targeted Optical Imaging Agents

In 2021, pafolacianine sodium (Cytalux) became the first FDA-approved receptor-targeted fluorescent imaging agent for intraoperative use, and many more are close to new drug application.[7] Pafolacianine is composed of a folic acid analogue bound to an NIR dye and targets folate-α (FRα) receptor-positive ovarian cancer.[7] The drug has the ability to localize to cancerous tissue within a few hours (1–3 hours) after infusion—this imaging timeframe is particularly helpful for surgeons in the application of FGS by allowing administration the day of surgery (an optimal imaging time of 6–12 hours is logistically very challenging).[31] Furthermore, its tumor-specific properties ensure rapid clearance from healthy tissue, minimizing undiscriminating fluorescence.[18,31]

The introduction of pafolacianine in FGS represents a profound step forward in oncological surgery. However, FDA approval of Cytalux as an intraoperative tumor-specific optical agent is limited to the cytoreduction of ovarian cancer.[7,32] As previously stated, up to 30% of HNC surgeries yield positive margins, which typically forecasts a poorer patient prognosis. Resection of HNC tumors can be particularly difficult because it is difficult to visualize differences between tumor and normal tissue during the deep portions of the resection and the relationship to critical unresectable structures in the surgical field.[5] Furthermore, taking an excessively wide margin results in poor functional outcomes. Therefore, the implementation of a disease-specific optical agent for HNC would be undoubtedly beneficial for patient outcome. As a clear demonstration of the rapid adoption of this technology by industry and the surgical community are currently 7 novel tumor-specific optical contrast agents being evaluated in HNC alone (**Table 1**).[25]

IDEAL DEVELOPMENT OF HEAD AND NECK CANCER-SPECIFIC FLUOROPHORES
Target Selection

The likelihood of finding biomarker expression that is universal to all head and neck tumor types remains a significant challenge.[18] However, researchers have developed a scoring system to evaluate the potential of a biomarker as a viable fluorophore target.[18,40] The Target Selection Criteria scoring system operates by reviewing 7 important characteristics of a suitable biomarker: (1) extracellular protein localization (to allow a circulating agent to bind), (2) diffuse upregulation through tumor tissue, (3) tumor-to-normal cell ratio greater than 10, (4) percentage of patients with overexpression, (5) previously imaged with success in vivo, (6) enzymatic activity, and (7) internalization (to allow accumulation beyond agent bound to the cell surface).[40] The maximum score that a cellular component can receive is 22, but a score of 18 is sufficient to signify a potential biomarker for tumor targeting purposes.[40] Currently, epidermal growth factor receptor (EGFR) is one of the most extensively studied

Table 1
Novel HNC specific FGS agents

Probe Name	Description	Fluorophore	Ligand Type	Clinical Trial Phase
Panitumumab-IRDye 800CW[33]	IV administration 1–5 d before surgery	IRDye-800	EGFR-targeting antibody	Phase 2
Cetuximab-IRDye80 0CW[34]	IV administration 4 d before surgery	IRDye-800	EGFR-targeting antibody	Phase 2
ABY-029[35]	Micro dose injection 1–3 h before surgery	IRDye-800	EGFR-targeting affibody	Phase 1
cRGDY-PEG-Cy5.5-C*[36]	Injected intratumorally before or during surgery	Cy5.5	Integrin-targeting silica nanoparticle	Phase 2
cRGD-ZW800–1[37]	Injected 4–24 h before surgery	ZW-800	Integrin-targeting silica nanoparticle	Phase 2
ONM-100[38]	IV administration on the day of surgery	ICG	pH-activated nanoparticle	Phase 2
PARPi-FL[39]	Applied topically for basal cell carcinoma	BODIPY-FL	PARP1-targeting small molecule	Phase 2

Abbreviations: EGFR, epidermal growth factor receptor; IV, intravenous; PARP1, poly(ADP-ribose) polymerase 1.

biomarkers in HNC.[41] EGFR is an attractive HNC target due to its high expression levels in malignant cells relative to normal tissue. Other head and neck targets currently being studied in clinical trials include integrin and poly(ADP-ribose) polymerase 1 (PARP1).[18]

Targeting Agent/Fluorophore

Most targeting ligands are small molecule-, peptide-, or antibody-based ligands; however, other ligand possibilities include affibodies, lectins and activatable ligands.[14,18] Cytalux contains a folate analogue ligand and is an example of a small molecule targeting agent.[14] At present, PARPi-FL—a small molecule probe that targets PARP1—is in phase 2 clinical trials for imaging of oral squamous cell carcinoma.[18,42] By virtue of their size, low-molecular-weight drug conjugates tend to exhibit faster pharmacokinetic properties, allowing for rapid contrast imaging ($\leq$ 1 hour postinfusion).[23,43] The disadvantage of rapidly cleared agents is that they have limited time to circulate through the tumor and although blood-borne background is lower, they have less time to accumulate in the tumor. Furthermore, with small ligands, the size of the fluorophore must be taken into consideration because it may affect binding, and as a result require complex synthesis requirements. Peptides are also considered targeting agents due to their high specificity and affinity to a broad range of receptors on malignant cell surfaces, paired with the advantages of being a relatively small ligand that can be renally cleared and usually have limited toxicity.[44] Antibody-based agents use the demarcating properties of immunoglobulins to target tumor-associated antigens on the cell surface; most were originally developed for immunotherapy, then later attached to contrast agents and used in subtherapeutic levels as a diagnostic tool for imaging.[14]

Activatable agents are unique in that they are optically inactive in their native state and upon enzymatic cleavage undergo activation and become visible by fluorescence imaging.[21] Activation by enzymatic cleavage is specific for tumors that have proteases concentrated at the peritumoral space.[45] Previously quenched fluorophores can, upon cleavage, demonstrate high levels of fluorescence.[18,21] Similarly are pH-sensitive agents that achieve activation through changes in pH (eg, ONM-100, a pH-sensitive ICG-based probe with a binary on/off mechanism).[38] Tumors tend to have an abnormally acidic extracellular environment due to their tendency to convert glucose to lactic acid. pH-sensitive dyes exploit this unique property of malignant cells and begin to fluoresce upon exposure to tumor.[46]

Because EGFR is currently the most extensively studied HNC biomarker, anti-EGFR antibodies—panitumumab and cetuximab—have received substantial attention in the development of head and neck-specific agents. As previously stated, NIR fluorophores exhibit ideal imaging results due to their high tissue penetration and low autofluorescence. Thus, dyes with absorption and emission peaks in this range are optimal for targeted optical imaging agents.[18,21,22] Both panitumumab and cetuximab have been conjugated to Li-Cor IRDye800CW, which fluoresces in the NIR range, and are undergoing phase 2 clinical trials.[25,35] Using repurposed therapeutic antibodies has the advantage of being safe and relatively inexpensive to manufacture, but they have limited commercial opportunities without support from the manufacturers of these agents.

Hardware

The ability of these optical agents to be successfully implemented in the clinic relies on the available instrument for visualization. As of 2020, there are 20 FDA-approved imaging devices for FGS. Because ICG is the most widely used fluorophore in FGS, most of the devices are tailored to ICG's emission peak (~800 nm) in the NIR range and are thus limited to capturing contrast agents with similar wavelengths.[25] At present, the most common imaging system for HNC FGS is the Stryker, the device is SPY-PHI, a portable handheld imager that captures an emission wavelength of ~825 nm. Following its FDA approval in 2005, many subsequent systems showed substantial similarities to the SPY-PHI.[26] Additional approved systems that capture fluorescent images in the NIR range—ideal for increased tissue penetration and low autofluorescence—include the Photodynamic Eye (PDE), Hamamatsu Photonics Co. (Hamamatsu, Japan), an ICG-detecting handheld device, and PINPOINT, Stryker, an endoscopic imaging device.[23]

Surgical Use Case

The implementation of tumor-specific optical agents in HNC surgeries is hugely impactful in tumor removal (in situ) and in evaluation of surgical margins (sentinel margins).[21] During tumor removal, intraoperative open-field fluorescence imaging can be used to detect second primary lesions, identify metastatic lymph nodes, and assess the extent of disease into nearby tissues (**Fig. 3**).[21] As previously stated, positive surgical margins are associated with increased local recurrence and a higher 5-year mortality rate among patients with HNC.[4] In a clinical trial evaluating panitumumab-IRDye800CW efficacy in FGS, it was determined that the accuracy of fluorescence intensity to identify the true sentinel margin was 96.4%, compared with the surgeon at 82.1%.[47] That is, immediately following tumor resection, ex vivo fluorescent molecular imaging of the resected tissue immediately improved the detection of positive margins.[48]

FUTURE OF THE FIELD
Robot-Assisted Head and Neck Cancer Surgery

Robotic surgery has become an increasingly popular intraoperative tool for HNC resection due to the technology's high precision and shortened patient postoperative

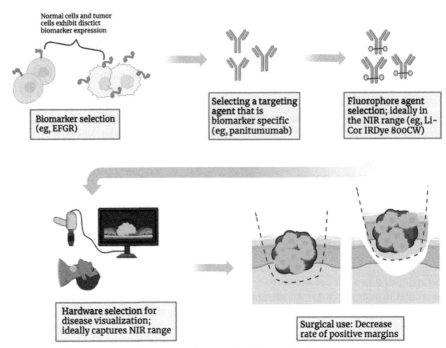

Fig. 3. Development and clinical translation of HNC-specific fluorophores. (Image created using BioRender.)

recovery time.[47] The da Vinci robot has dominated the robotic surgical system market since its first FDA approval in 2000.[49] After the da Vinci system was cleared for transoral robotic surgery in 2009, it was rapidly adopted by head and neck surgical oncologists, particularly because it helped surgeons manage cases with difficult-to-access tumors.[50] In 2011, the FDA approved fluorescence imaging of ICG in surgical robots. The device was marketed as the da Vinci Fluorescence Vision Imaging System—later renamed da Vinci Firefly—as an adjunctive tool to the da Vinci Si Surgical System Intuitive Surgical (Sunnyvale, CA).[51] Because this robot is uniquely tailored to ICG imaging, it is limited by the nonspecificity of this fluorescent agent. The da Vinci robot eliminates surgeon access to tactile feedback; thus, visual dependence on a nonspecific dye can yield an incomplete evaluation of the surgical field.[47] However, recent advancements in this imaging device address these concerns; the Advanced Firefly is not limited to ICG and can capture a wider range of optical agents. One study found that, after preoperative administration of panitumumab-IRDYE800 in patients with HNC, the Advanced Firefly allowed for better intraoperative delineation of tumor margins, demonstrating the heightened potential of robot-assisted HNC resections.[52]

Beyond Fluorescence

Although this review primarily focuses on fluorescence-based imaging, advances in intraoperative imaging techniques are not limited to this signaling modality. For example, the concept of radioguided surgery—which requires the preoperative administration of radiolabeled tracers—was developed approximately 70 years ago. Following preoperative injection, radionuclides emit gamma photons, which are detected by a gamma detection probe system.[53] Although intraoperative use of radiotracers for HNC has been primarily confined to radioguided SLN biopsy, there has been increased interest in developing tumor-seeking procedures that use both radioguidance and fluorescence-based guidance for enhanced visualization of meta-static disease.[54] Use of radionuclides is synergistic with fluorescent agents. Radionu-clides have deeper tissue penetration compared with fluorescent agents, but lower resolution. In contrast, fluorescent agents have very high resolution but limited depth penetration. Thus, accurate detection of disease may require combined application— much like the current standard of care in sentinel node biopsy. The administration of [111]Ind-panitumumab for preoperative and intraoperative identification of metastatic disease of the head and neck is being explored in clinical trials (NCT04840472). As FGS continues to develop in the HNC field, the paired utilization of fluorophores and radiotracers may be the next step forward for optimal intraoperative imaging.

SUMMARY

For decades, head and neck surgical oncologists have relied on preoperative anatom-ical imaging (PET, CT, and MRI), intraoperative visual and tactile cues, and FSA for tu-mor resection. These methods have yielded a stagnant and high rate ($\sim$30%) of positive surgical margins in HNCs, indicating a need for improved intraoperative visu-alization of malignant disease.[5,21]

The rapid emergence of FGS in the past 10 years has provided surgeons with a mo-lecular imaging modality with real-time intraoperative feedback. Excitement for devel-oping agents for other tumor types has been propelled by recent FDA approval of Cytalux, an FRα-targeting fluorophore agent, marking a monumental step forward in intraoperative oncological treatment. Although Cytalux is currently only approved for ovarian cancer treatment, its approval lends support to the need for intraoperative tar-geting agents.[7,21] Ongoing development and testing of head and neck-specific fluo-rescent agents paired with advancements in NIR imaging software and hardware (eg, Advanced Firefly) ultimately illuminates the potential for FGS in the head and neck field.

CLINICS CARE POINTS

- More than 30 clinical trials are currently investigating tumor-specific agents and one was recently FDA approved.

- Optical imaging agents for FGS are complementary to current anatomic and metabolic imaging modalities used for preoperative evaluation.

- Surgeons will need to become familiar with the capabilities and limitations such as safety, depth of imaging, and clinical applications.

- Depth of penetration of these fluorescent agents is limited to 1 to 2 cm and therefore can only be used in the intraoperative setting and require specialized hardware for imaging.

DISCLOSURE

The authors have nothing to disclose.

REFERENCES

1. Vigneswaran N, Williams MD. Epidemiologic trends in head and neck cancer and aids in diagnosis. Oral Maxillofac Surg Clin North Am 2014;26:123–41.

2. Pollock NI, Grandis JR. HER2 as a therapeutic target in head and neck squamous cell carcinoma. Clin Cancer Res 2015;21:526–33.

3. Eldeeb H, Macmillan C, Elwell C, et al. The effect of the surgical margins on the outcome of patients with head and neck squamous cell carcinoma: single institution experience. Cancer Biol Med 2012;9:29–33.

4. Li MM, Puram SV, Silverman DA, et al. Margin analysis in head and neck cancer: state of the art and future directions. Ann Surg Oncol 2019;26:4070–80.

5. van Keulen S, Nishio N, Fakurnejad S, et al. Intraoperative tumor assessment using real-time molecular imaging in head and neck cancer patients. J Am Coll Surg 2019;229:560–7.e561.

6. Mieog JSD, Achterberg FB, Zlitni A, et al. Fundamentals and developments in fluorescence-guided cancer surgery. Nat Rev Clin Oncol 2022;19:9–22.

7. Tanyi JL, Chon HS, Morgan MA, et al. Phase 3, randomized, single-dose, open-label study to investigate the safety and efficacy of pafolacianine sodium injection (OTL38) for intraoperative imaging of folate receptor positive ovarian cancer. J Clin Oncol 2021;39:5503.

8. Patel PR, De Jesus O. StatPearls. StatPearls Publishing Copyright © 2022, StatPearls Publishing LLC.; 2022.

9. Hamilton B. In: Bryan Bell R, Fernandes RP, Andersen PE, editors. Oral, head and neck oncology and reconstructive surgery. Elsevier; 2018. p. 107–18.

10. Hoffmann EJ, Phelps ME, Mullani NA, et al. Design and performance characteristics of a whole-body positron transaxial tomograph. J Nucl Med 1976;17:493–502.

11. Fletcher JW, Djulbegovic B, Soares HP, et al. Recommendations on the Use of ^{18}F-FDG PET in oncology. J Nucl Med 2008;49:480.

12. Griffeth LK. Use of PET/CT scanning in cancer patients: technical and practical considerations. Proc (Bayl Univ Med Cent) 2005;18:321–30.

13. Kapoor V, McCook BM, Torok FS. An Introduction to PET-CT Imaging. RadioGraphics 2004;24:523–43.

14. Joshi BP, Wang TD. Targeted optical imaging agents in cancer: focus on clinical applications. Contrast Media Mol Imaging 2018;2015237. https://doi.org/10.1155/2018/2015237.

15. Campbell S. A short history of sonography in obstetrics and gynaecology. Facts Views Vis Obgyn 2013;5:213–29.

16. Wang X, Yang M. The application of ultrasound image in cancer diagnosis. J Healthc Eng 2021;2021:8619251.

17. Carovac A, Smajlovic F, Junuzovic D. Application of ultrasound in medicine. Acta Inform Med 2011;19:168–71.

18. de Boer E, Harlaar NJ, Taruttis A, et al. Optical innovations in surgery. Br J Surg 2015;102:e56–72.

19. Stewart HL, Birch DJS. Fluorescence guided surgery. Methods Appl Fluorescence 2021;9:042002.

20. Gioux S, Choi HS, Frangioni JV. Image-guided surgery using invisible near-infrared light: fundamentals of clinical translation. Mol Imaging 2010;9:237–55.

21. Lee YJ, Krishnan G, Nishio N, et al. Intraoperative fluorescence-guided surgery in head and neck squamous cell carcinoma. Laryngoscope 2021;131:529–34.

22. Schaafsma BE, Mieog JSD, Hutteman M, et al. The clinical use of indocyanine green as a near-infrared fluorescent contrast agent for image-guided oncologic surgery. J Surg Oncol 2011;104:323–32.

23. Zhang RR, Schroeder AB, Grudzinski JJ, et al. Beyond the margins: real-time detection of cancer using targeted fluorophores. Nat Rev Clin Oncol 2017;14: 347–64.

24. Crawford KL, Pacheco FV, Lee Y-J, et al. A scoping review of ongoing fluorescence-guided surgery clinical trials in otolaryngology. Laryngoscope 2022;132: 36–44.

25. Barth CW, Gibbs SL. Fluorescence image-guided surgery - a perspective on contrast agent development. Proc SPIE Int Soc Opt Eng 2020;11222:112220J.

26. van Manen L, Handgraaf HJM, Diana M, et al. A practical guide for the use of indocyanine green and methylene blue in fluorescence-guided abdominal surgery. J Surg Oncol 2018;118:283–300.

27. Fetzer S, Holmes S. Relieving the pain of sentinel lymph node biopsy tracer injection. Clin J Oncol Nurs 2008;12:668–70.

28. Hadjipanayis CG, Stummer W. 5-ALA and FDA approval for glioma surgery. J Neurooncol 2019;141:479–86.

29. Malmström P-U, Hedelin H, Thomas YK, et al. Fluorescence-guided transurethral resection of bladder cancer using hexaminolevulinate: analysis of health economic impact in Sweden. Scand J Urol Nephrol 2009;43:192–8.

30. Zhou H, Gao Y, Liu Y, et al. Targeted fluorescent imaging of a novel FITC-labeled PSMA ligand in prostate cancer. Amino Acids 2022;54:147–55.

31. Mahalingam SM, Kularatne SA, Myers CH, et al. Evaluation of novel tumor-targeted near-infrared probe for fluorescence-guided surgery of cancer. J Med Chem 2018;61:9637–46.

32. de la Torre BG, Albericio F. The Pharmaceutical Industry in 2021. An Analysis of FDA Drug Approvals from the Perspective of Molecules. Molecules 2022;27. https://doi.org/10.3390/molecules27031075.

33. Heath CH, Deep NL, Sweeny L, et al. Use of panitumumab-IRDye800 to image microscopic head and neck cancer in an orthotopic surgical model. Ann Surg Oncol 2012;19:3879–87.

34. Gao RW, Teraphongphom N, de Boer E, et al. Safety of panitumumab-IRDye800CW and cetuximab-IRDye800CW for fluorescence-guided surgical navigation in head and neck cancers. Theranostics 2018;8:2488–95.

35. Samkoe KS, Gunn JR, Marra K, et al. Toxicity and pharmacokinetic profile for single-dose injection of ABY-029: a fluorescent Anti-EGFR synthetic affibody molecule for human use. Mol Imaging Biol 2017;19:512–21.

36. Sun Y, Zeng X, Xiao Y, et al. Novel dual-function near-infrared II fluorescence and PET probe for tumor delineation and image-guided surgery. Chem Sci 2018;9: 2092–7.

37. Handgraaf HJM, Boonstra MC, Prevoo HAJM, et al. Real-time near-infrared fluorescence imaging using cRGD-ZW800-1 for intraoperative visualization of multiple cancer types. Oncotarget 2017;8:21054–66.

38. Witjes M, Voskuil F, Steinkamp P, et al. Fluorescence guided surgery using the pH-activated micellar tracer ONM-100: first-in-human proof of principle in head and neck squamous cell carcinoma. J Oral Maxillofacial Surg 2019;77:e38. https://doi.org/10.1016/j.joms.2019.06.061.

39. Irwin CP, Portorreal Y, Brand C, et al. PARPi-FL–a fluorescent PARP1 inhibitor for glioblastoma imaging. Neoplasia 2014;16:432–40.

40. van Oosten M, Crane LM, Bart J, et al. Selecting potential targetable biomarkers for imaging purposes in colorectal cancer using target selection criteria (TASC): a novel target identification tool. Transl Oncol 2011;4:71–82.

41. Bossi P, Resteghini C, Paielli N, et al. Prognostic and predictive value of EGFR in head and neck squamous cell carcinoma. Oncotarget 2016;7:74362–79.
42. Kossatz S, Brand C, Gutiontov S, et al. Detection and delineation of oral cancer with a PARP1 targeted optical imaging agent. Sci Rep 2016;6:21371.
43. Srinivasarao M, Galliford CV, Low PS. Principles in the design of ligand-targeted cancer therapeutics and imaging agents. Nat Rev Drug Discov 2015;14:203–19.
44. Becker A, Hessenius C, Licha K, et al. Receptor-targeted optical imaging of tumors with near-infrared fluorescent ligands. Nat Biotechnol 2001;19:327–31.
45. Whitley MJ, Cardona DM, Lazarides AL, et al. A mouse-human phase 1 co-clinical trial of a protease-activated fluorescent probe for imaging cancer. Sci Transl Med 2016;8:320ra324.
46. Steinkamp P, Voskuil F, van der Vegt B, et al. Metabolic acidosis in cancer: a new strategy using a ph activated imaging agent for fluorescence-guided surgery in humans. Eur J Surg Oncol 2020;46:e163–4. https://doi.org/10.1016/j.ejso.2019.11.433.
47. Gorpas D, Phipps J, Bec J, et al. Autofluorescence lifetime augmented reality as a means for real-time robotic surgery guidance in human patients. Scientific Rep 2019;9:1187.
48. Krishnan G, van den Berg NS, Nishi N, et al. Fluorescent molecular imaging can improve intraoperative sentinel margin detection in oral squamous cell carcinoma. J Nucl Med 2022;121:262235.
49. Leal Ghezzi T, Campos Corleta O. 30 years of robotic surgery. World J Surg 2016;40:2550–7.
50. Couey M, Patel A, Bell RB. In: Acero J, editor. Innovations and new developments in craniomaxillofacial reconstruction. Springer International Publishing; 2021. p. 199–210.
51. Lee Y-J, van den Berg NS, Orosco RK, et al. A narrative review of fluorescence imaging in robotic-assisted surgery. Laparosc Surg 2021;5:31.
52. Rao, S., Stone, L.D., Jeyarajan H. et al., Standardized Fluorescence-Guided TORS Using An Integrated Signal Source. Poster presented at: The AHNS Annual Meeting; April 27-28, 2022; Dallas, TX.
53. Povoski SP, Neff RL, Mojzisik CM, et al. A comprehensive overview of radio-guided surgery using gamma detection probe technology. World J Surg Oncol 2009;7:11.
54. Mariani G, Valdés Olmos RA, Vidal-Sicart S, et al. Radioguided surgery. J Nucl Med 2021;62:591.

Contrast-Enhanced Intraoperative Ultrasound of the Liver

Gloria Y. Chang, MD[a], David T. Fetzer, MD[b],
Matthew R. Porembka, MD[c],*

KEYWORDS

- HCC • CRLM • Ultrasound • Contrast-enhanced • Cirrhosis • Liver
- Focal liver lesions

KEY POINTS

- The safety profile of ultrasound contrast agents and real-time acquisition of dynamic enhancement patterns of liver lesions intraoperatively confers valuable added benefit over traditional liver imaging modalities such as computed tomography, MRI, and grayscale intraoperative ultrasound.
- Contrast-enhanced intraoperative ultrasound (CE-IOUS) is useful for distinguishing hepatocellular carcinoma from benign lesions in patients with cirrhosis in whom nodules detected on grayscale IOUS may appear indeterminate.
- CE-IOUS can improve the sensitivity of liver metastases detection for patients with colorectal liver metastasis, even if gadoxetate disodium enhanced magnetic resonance imaging (Gd-EOB-MRI) has already been performed.

INTRODUCTION

Intraoperative ultrasonography (IOUS) is an accurate and sensitive diagnostic technique that has become standard of care in liver surgery. Although IOUS can identify lesions and help direct surgical planning by defining anatomic relationships, IOUS falls short in 2 main areas. Focal liver lesions (FLL), particularly in cirrhotic livers, can be difficult to distinguish as benign or malignant with grayscale IOUS alone. Additionally, in the setting of colorectal cancer with liver metastases (CRLM), small metastatic foci may still be missed. With the development of ultrasound contrast agents (UCA), the use of contrast-enhanced ultrasonography (CEUS) both in and out of the operating

^a Division of Surgical Oncology, Department of Surgery, University of Texas Southwestern Medical Center, 5323 Harry Hines Boulevard, Dallas, TX 75390, USA; ^b Department of Radiology, University of Texas Southwestern Medical Center, 5323 Harry Hines Boulevard, E6-230-BF, Dallas, TX 75390-9316, USA; ^c Division of Surgical Oncology, Department of Surgery, Dedman Family Scholar in Clinical Care, University of Texas Southwestern Medical Center, 5323 Harry Hines Boulevard, NB2.340, Dallas, TX 75390, USA
* Corresponding author.
E-mail address: matthew.porembka@utsouthwestern.edu

Surg Oncol Clin N Am 31 (2022) 707–719
https://doi.org/10.1016/j.soc.2022.06.007

Abbreviations	
CEUS	contrast-enhanced ultrasound
CE-IOUS	contrast-enhanced intraoperative ultrasound
CRLM	colorectal liver metastasis
CT	computed tomography
DLM	disappearing liver metastasis
FLL	focal liver lesion
HCC	hepatocellular carcinoma
IOUS	intraoperative ultrasound
LI-RADS	Liver Imaging Reporting and Data System
MRI	magnetic resonance imaging
MI	mechanical index
UCA	ultrasound contrast agent

room has allowed for more sensitive detection and accurate characterization of FLLs. In this review, the basic principles of contrast-enhanced intraoperative ultrasound (CE-IOUS) and characteristic imaging examples are reviewed. The main indications for liver CE-IOUS and the data comparing this technique with other imaging modalities are also described.

EVOLUTION OF LIVER IMAGING

The initial detection and characterization of FLLs is important for accurate diagnosis and appropriate management. With its widespread availability, contrast-enhanced computed tomography (CE-CT) is routinely obtained. However, with improved resolution, contrast-enhanced MRI (CE-MRI) has become the gold standard, particularly for smaller lesions. MRI using liver-specific contrast agents such as gadoxetate disodium (Gd-EOB-MRI) adds improved sensitivity for metastases and specificity for primary liver lesions. Although each of these imaging modalities play an important role in the evaluation of FLLs, once the decision is made to proceed with surgery, ultrasound remains a critical intraoperative tool.

Previously, the intraoperative assessment of the liver was limited to direct visualization and palpation, severely limiting the understanding of internal anatomy. Initial reports primarily out of Japan by Makuuchi in the 1970s describing intraoperative ultrasound (IOUS) for performing subsegmentectomies were followed by rapid dissemination.[1,2] IOUS is the standard of care in liver surgery and used to identify lesions, delineate anatomy, and plan resection.

With the advent of ultrasound contrast agents (UCA), real-time ultrasound characterization of FLLs has become possible. The use of UCAs started in the 1960s, initially with agitated saline with echocardiography.[3] SonoVue/Lumason (Bracco Diagnostics, Monroe Township, NJ) was approved by Food and Drug Administration (FDA) for liver imaging in both children and adults in 2016. The use of this agent, along with several others, has been published widely. Indications for CEUS include characterization of indeterminate lesions on previous imaging or if a contrast study is required though contrast-enhanced CT or MRI are contraindicated. CEUS has also had an expanding role in various interventional radiology procedures such as percutaneous biopsy, tumor ablation, and transarterial chemoembolization, where its use can improve procedural guidance and provide valuable preprocedure and postprocedure assessments to evaluate treatment response.[4] As transabdominal CEUS has gained traction as a useful diagnostic and potentially therapeutic modality, its use was slowly transitioned into the operating room.[5]

CE-IOUS carries various benefits and drawbacks that overlap with those of transabdominal CEUS (**Table 1**). Some practical advantages of CEUS include the ability to

Table 1	
Benefits and drawbacks of contrast-enhanced intraoperative ultrasound of the liver	
Benefit	**Drawback**
• No ionizing radiation • No nephrotoxicity or hepatotoxicity associated with UCA; no need for prior renal or hepatic function laboratory testing • Dynamic enhancement characterization of newly detected lesions or lesions that are indeterminate on CT, MRI, and/or IOUS • Real-time imaging allows for practitioner to ensure appropriate timing of contrast • Ability to perform repeat contrasted imaging for the same or new lesions • Immediate imaging and interpretation may provide valuable information that can impact surgical decision-making	• Associated upfront costs for obtaining the appropriate equipment, software, contrast agents, and systems in place • Operator dependent; initial learning curve to become familiar with the equipment, the technical aspects of performing the exam, and the accurate interpretation of real-time images • The volume and diversity of cases need to be sufficient to maintain adequate practitioner skills • The addition of intraoperative time as a result of additional imaging studies • Other drawbacks that are inherent to ultrasound: risk of missed lesions due to operator-dependent manual scanning of liver, difficult to reach areas, poor penetration of lesions deeper lesions

obtain contrast-enhanced imaging of lesions using UCA in patients with renal failure or those with allergies to iodinated-based or gadolinium-based contrast; capture temporal enhancement patterns of lesions in real time, thereby eliminating the potential for ambiguous image interpretation due to poor contrast timing; and acquire imaging for those with MRI-incompatible implanted devices or foreign bodies.[6]

CONTRAST-ENHANCED ULTRASOUND
Basic Principles of Contrast-Enhanced Ultrasound

Getting started
Implementation of a CE-IOUS program may require institutional approval by safety, pharmacology, and therapeutics committees and acquisition of separate CEUS supplies in addition to the standard ultrasound equipment. Contrast-specific ultrasound machine software may need to be purchased and equipment optimized for CEUS. SonoVue (Bracco Diagnostics Inc., Milan, Italy) is currently the only commercially available UCA approved for liver imaging. Specialized training in both the technical aspects of CEUS and the interpretation of the dynamic enhanced images that are obtained during the procedure is recommended.[7]

Ultrasound contrast agent
UCA are composed of small particles: gas-filled microbubbles stabilized by a lipid or protein biological shell. Each microbubble is slightly smaller than a red blood cell, although too large to pass through the vascular endothelium into the interstitium, allowing them to act as pure blood pool agents. They allow for enhancement of both microvasculature and macrovasculature and can effectively be used to highlight characteristic enhancement patterns of lesions during the various vascular phases of the liver.

There are several contrast agents available for liver imaging including SonoVue/Lumason (sulfur hexafluoride lipid Type A microspheres, stabilized by a phospholipid shell), Definity/Luminity (octafluoropane with a lipid shell, Lantheus Medical Imaging, Inc., North Billerica, MA, USA), and Sonazoid (perfluorobutane also with a phospholipid shell, GE Healthcare, Oslo, Norway).[8] Sonazoid is unique because its negative charge encourages uptake by Kupffer cells and will demonstrate an additional "postvascular" or "Kupffer phase" that starts at 10 minutes after contrast injection and lasts for an hour or more (similar to the hepatobiliary phase in Gd-EOB-MRI).[9] Malignant liver lesions typically lack Kupffer cells and will therefore seem hypoechoic during the Kupffer phase, whereas normal liver parenchyma will remain enhanced.[3]

The UCA is typically injected via a peripheral vein, although central venous catheters may also be used. Once in circulation, the microbubbles will oscillate in the presence of an ultrasound pulse and produce a nonlinear response. Because the surrounding tissue predominantly responds in a linear fashion, contrast-specific software can separate the nonlinear signal specifically received from microbubbles, allowing for a "contrast-only" image.[10] The degree of the nonlinear frequency produced is dependent on the transmit frequency of the ultrasound system. Signal can be increased by increasing the system's output power; however, this increases the mechanical index (MI). The MI is an estimate of the maximum amplitude of the pressure pulse in tissue and reflects the likelihood to cause cavitation. Higher MI corresponds to higher acoustic pressure and therefore more rapid microbubble destruction. Generally, low MI (<0.3) is used for most CE-IOUS.[11]

UCA are safe. They have not been shown to be nephrotoxic or hepatotoxic and therefore do not require any renal or hepatic function testing before injection. Side effects are uncommon and generally mild when they do occur. Serious events are extremely rare with a reported rate of 0.001% with no deaths or life-threatening anaphylactic reactions.[12–14] UCAs are cleared quickly with a half-life of 6 minutes for Sonovue and 1.3 minutes for Definity, allowing for multiple injections during a single examination. The gas core of the microbubbles will diffuse through the shell and be eliminated by respiration while the shell is metabolized in the lipid pool by the liver.[15]

Instruments

An ultrasound machine with contrast-specific software using a low MI (<0.3) and optimized presets for use of UCAs is required to perform CE-IOUS. A variety of transducers including a linear, convex T, or finger probe can be used, although a curvilinear array may be most preferred for liver imaging using UCAs as microbubbles oscillate best at lower frequencies. The gain should be set just above the noise floor such that the contrast image initially appears black with a very low level of noise. The focus should be set just deep to the lesion of interest because more microbubble destruction will occur right at the focal zone.[11]

A split screen format is generally utilized with one screen displaying the contrast image and the second displaying a reconstructed conventional B-mode image simultaneously (**Fig. 1**). Because the contrast-enhanced image will initially appear black, the second B-mode screen allows the machine operator to confirm adequate positioning of the probe and that the lesion of interest remains in the field of view during scanning.[11,16]

Protocol

After adequate liver mobilization and manual palpation, systematic IOUS in B-mode of the entire liver is performed to look for new nodules, confirm previously diagnosed lesions, and identify major vascular and biliary anatomy to establish surgical strategy. If any lesions requiring further characterization are encountered, CE-IOUS is performed.[10]

After preparation, the appropriate dose of the agent is injected (FDA-approved dose of 2.4 mL for SonoVue/Lumason) through a peripheral vein (at least 20 gauge and no

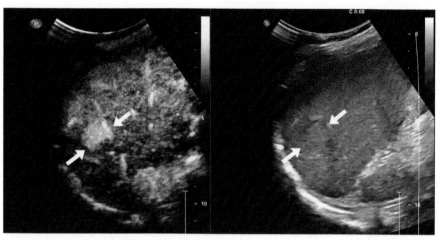

Fig. 1. Typical split screen format with B-mode image on one side (*right*) and contrast-enhanced image on the other (*left*). Contrast-enhanced image demonstrates arterial phase hyperenhancement of an HCC nodule indicated by the arrows in a 65-year-old woman with history of hepatitis C cirrhosis.

IV-line filters) followed by a 5 to 10 mL saline flush. A 3-way stopcock is helpful to facilitate rapid administration of contrast and saline injections, particularly if multiple doses are expected.[11] Because high pressure and turbulent flow can cause microbubble destruction, the injections are performed over several seconds and in axis with the vein.[3,11] A timer on the ultrasound system and cine clip recording are started after the contrast injection.

The 3 vascular phases include the arterial phase (starting at 20–30 seconds), portal venous phase (30 seconds to 2 minutes), and late phase (2 to 5 minutes). The microbubbles should begin to come into view 20 seconds or less after contrast injection, marking the start of the arterial phase. The lesion should be imaged continuously until peak arterial phase enhancement is reached to capture the "wash in" pattern. To minimize microbubble destruction, the lesion can then be scanned intermittently (every 30 seconds) during the portal venous to late phases until the microbubbles have cleared from the circulation (up to 4–6 minutes).[16]

If the lesion is incompletely characterized with the first injection or if additional lesions require contrast-enhanced scanning, repeat contrast injection can be performed after enough time has passed for most microbubbles to have cleared from the liver (about 10 minutes for SonoVue; greater than 1 hour for Sonazoid). Conventional B-mode scanning (higher MI) can also be used during this time to facilitate more rapid microbubble destruction.[11]

Indications

Hepatocellular carcinoma

Although routine preoperative imaging with high-resolution CT or MRI provides vital information for identifying nodules and determining resectability, the sensitivity, particularly for small lesions (<1 cm), remains low.[17] IOUS is an essential tool in hepatic resections for hepatocellular carcinoma (HCC) in order to identify known and occult tumor nodules and to define their relationship to vital hepatic structures. However, while IOUS improves the detection of nodules in cirrhotic livers, IOUS can also overestimate tumor staging because 70% to 80% of detected nodules detected on IOUS are regenerative, dysplastic, or otherwise benign.[18-20] Although intraoperative biopsy can be considered, it is not preferred due to a high false-negative rate.[21] CE-IOUS can evaluate the vascularity and enhancement patterns of lesions detected on grayscale IOUS in real time to help differentiate benign nodules from HCC.[5,22]

HCC shares similar enhancement characteristics during CE-IOUS as in CE-CT or CE-MRI: HCC will hyperenhance during the arterial phase, and subsequently show washout, appearing hypoechoic in the portal venous or late phases. In contrast, in a cirrhotic liver, regenerative and dysplastic nodules will typically seem isoenhancing in all phases. In 2016, the American College of Radiology endorsed the CEUS Liver Imaging Reporting and Data System, which provides a classification system for interpreting CEUS and determining the likelihood of HCC in at risk patients.[16] The scoring system ranges from LR-1 (definitively benign) to LR-5 (definitively malignant). Although this schema applies specifically to extracorporeal CEUS, the general enhancement patterns described are consistent with those seen in CE-IOUS. A separate classification system for enhancement patterns seen specifically with CE-IOUS in cirrhotic patients has also been described by Torzilli and colleagues.[19] (**Figs. 2–4**).

Multiple studies have reported on the utility of CE-IOUS using SonoVue in detecting HCC at hepatectomy. The first report demonstrating feasibility of using CE-IOUS demonstrated that new information was obtained in 9 of 20 patients where new information included the detection of additional nodules not seen on previous preoperative imaging or conventional IOUS that were later determined to be malignant.[5] A subsequent series of 87 patients with HCC undergoing hepatectomy reported a 100% sensitivity and 69% specificity for CE-IOUS with 25% undergoing modified operative plan based on CE-IOUS.[19]

CE-IOUS with Sonazoid for hepatic resection for HCC is also well described. Because Sonazoid will accumulate in Kupffer cells, which malignant lesions notably lack, an additional "postvascular" or Kupffer phase imaging can differentiate

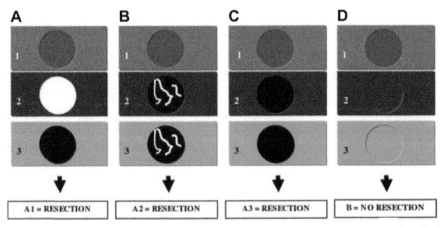

Fig. 2. Schema with classification of various liver nodule enhancement patterns as described by Torzilli and colleagues[19] (*A*) Fully enhanced nodule in arterial phase (2) and unenhanced in late phases (3). (*B*) Nodule demonstrates intramodular neovascularization in arterial phase (2) and persists through late phases (3). (*C*) Unenhanced nodule in both arterial (2) and late phases (3). (*D*) Isoenhancing nodule throughout all phases. (*From* Torzilli G, Palmisano A, Del Fabbro D, et al. Contrast-enhanced intraoperative ultrasonography during surgery for hepatocellular carcinoma in liver cirrhosis: is it useful or useless? A prospective cohort study of our experience. *Ann Surg Oncol.* 2007;14(4):1347-1355. https://doi.org/10.1245/s10434-006-9278-3.)

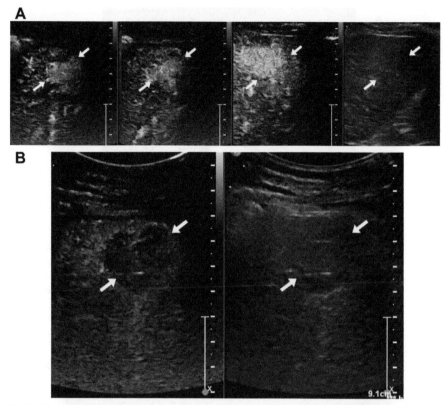

Fig. 3. Hepatocellular carcinoma. A 62-year-old man with history of hepatitis B, cirrhosis, and prior TACE for HCC. (*A*) HCC nodule (indicated by arrows) demonstrating progressive arterial phase hyperenhancement on CEUS. (*B*) Same nodule demonstrating delayed washout during portal venous phase, characteristic of HCC.

malignant from benign lesions. Sonazoid is currently approved for use only in Japan, Norway, Korea, Singapore, Taiwan, and China, with most literature reflecting increasing use in Asia. Multiple studies in HCC patients demonstrate sensitivities of 65% to 98%, specificities of 83% to 94%.[23–25]

Studies directly comparing Sonazoid and SonoVue as comparative UCA for CE-IOUS are largely lacking. Preliminary studies comparing the 2 agents for CEUS outside the operating room have demonstrated Sonazoid to be noninferior to SonoVue in diagnosing FLL as benign or malignant.[14,26]

Colorectal liver metastases

Among those with colorectal cancer, 25% to 30% will develop metastatic disease in the liver in the first 5 years of disease.[27] For CRLM, hepatic resection of all visible disease is the primary treatment option that offers long-term survival. Although curative-intent surgical resection of CRLM is considered the gold-standard treatment, it remains characterized by a high recurrence rate (64%) with most patients recurring within 1 year.[28,29] Because potential sites of persistent disease can lead to incomplete resection and early recurrence, more sensitive detection of CRLM is needed. UCA with IOUS can identify additional sites of metastatic disease. With CE-IOUS, these lesions seem to de-enhance during the portal venous and late

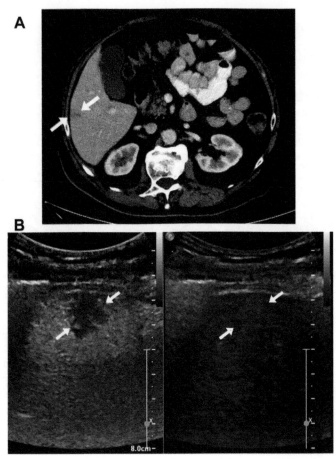

Fig. 4. Colorectal liver metastasis. A 68-year-old man with history of diffuse large B-cell lymphoma who presented with new biopsy proven rectal adenocarcinoma. Staging abdominal CT demonstrated new low density, ill-defined liver mass (indicated by arrows) (*A*). Subsequent CEUS revealed marked rapid washout with clear delineation of the corresponding lesion at 4 minutes, consistent with metastatic disease (*B*).

phases (early washout) and are similarly hypoechoic during the postvascular phase with Sonazoid injection.

CE-IOUS has been shown to be more sensitive than conventional grayscale ultrasound and may detect up to 10% to 15% additional CRLMs.[30] A systematic review and meta-analysis by Liu and colleagues including 13 studies evaluating the diagnostic performance of CE-IOUS for CRLM found CE-IOUS to be the most sensitive modality available for the detection of CRLM. With a total of 682 patients and 2,303 liver lesions, they reported a pooled sensitivity of 94% (range 89%–97%) and a pooled specificity of 82% (range 62%–93%) for CE-IOUS. This was compared with the pooled sensitivity and specificity of MRI (85% and 82%, respectively), IOUS (80% and 93%, respectively), and preoperative imaging (CT/MRI; 77% and 88%, respectively).[31]

A second meta-analysis examining CE-IOUS for CRLM similarly found CE-IOUS to be superior over CT, MRI, and IOUS in its sensitivity and accuracy. Among those who had new CRLM identified by CE-IOUS, surgical decision-making was affected in 51.8%,

71% of whom underwent more extensive hepatectomy and 11.7% were deemed nonoperable.[30] In a separate prospective single-institution clinical trial examining 47 patients with high tumor load, IOUS/CE-IOUS changed operative strategy in 35% of patients due to detection of additional hepatic lesions by IOUS (25%) or CEIOUS (10%).[32]

Disappearing liver metastasis. With the increasing use and efficacy of preoperative chemotherapy for CRLM, detection of liver metastases can be made even more challenging. Chemotherapy-induced liver damage and resulting steatosis can make lesions more difficult to distinguish on repeat imaging. Moreover, chemotherapy can result in "disappearing liver metastases" (DLM) or malignant lesions previously seen on imaging that demonstrate complete radiologic response on repeat cross-sectional imaging. Although DLMs may no longer be visible on standard preoperative imaging, complete pathological response may not necessarily be achieved. A focus of residual microscopic disease may persist with 59% to 78% reportedly reappearing in situ.[33] There are varying approaches to DLMs with many resecting only the disease that remains visible, whereas others resect original sites of disease.[34] In a circumstance in which resection of all disease is required for a chance at cure, the need for sensitive detection of all foci of disease is paramount.

Advances in imaging, particularly with liver-specific contrast-enhanced MRI (Gd-EOB-MRI), have improved the detection of malignant liver lesions that were previously too small to be detected. Both transabdominal CEUS and Gd-EOB-MRI have been separately found to be superior to CE-CT.[35–37] Studies comparing CEUS with Gd-EOB-MRI have had varying results, although most finding Gd-EOB-MRI to ultimately be more sensitive of the two.[35,38,39]

Additional studies comparing the intraoperative use of CEUS with Gd-EOB-MRI have been separately reported. A meta-analysis comparing the diagnostic performance of imaging modalities in detecting true pathologic response in patients with DLMs after chemotherapy found Gd-EOB-MRI or CE-IOUS to be the most accurate with negative predictive values of 0.73 and 0.79, respectively, compared with CT, PET, and IOUS (0.47, 0.22, 0.54, respectively). Given the intraoperative nature of CE-IOUS, MRI is the most appropriate imaging modality for the detection of DLM after chemotherapy, and reimaging with Gd-EOB-MRI is recommended before further surgical decision-making if preoperative imaging demonstrates DLM.[34]

Several studies have reported on the added utility of CE-IOUS using Sonazoid even if Gd-EOB-MRI is performed. Oba and colleagues[40] reported the detection rates of DLMs in patients with colorectal liver metastases after chemotherapy following sequential use of Gd-EOB-MRI and CE-IOUS using Sonazoid. Sensitivity of preoperative Gd-EOB-MRI alone was 48%, which increased to a sensitivity of 93% with the addition of CE-IOUS. In a separate study comparing the use of CE-IOUS using Sonazoid, Gd-EOB-MRI, CE-CT, and CEUS in the detection of DLM, CE-IOUS was the most sensitive, newly identifying additional CRLMs in 16% and modifying the planned surgical procedure in 14% of the patients.[41]

Ultimately, CE-CT remains the most widespread and accessible for the initial detection and characterization of liver lesions. The subsequent use of one or a combination of Gd-EOB-MRI, CEUS, and CE-IOUS will depend on careful patient selection and the availability of the various imaging modalities.

POINTERS AND PITFALLS

CE-IOUS can detect new lesions and provide additional information on previously seen lesions. It confers the benefit of real-time, continuous contrasted imaging as opposed to snapshots taken at predetermined time points that rely on accurate contrast timing, as with CE-CT or CE-MRI. Additionally, the unique characteristics of UCAs make them safe to use without the risk of hepatic or renal toxicity, all while avoiding any radiation exposure.

However, CE-IOUS has several drawbacks. Lesions in hard to access areas of the liver such as segment VIII or subdiaphragmatic areas may be overlooked. Additionally, given the recency of UCA approval and availability in the United States, the required equipment and contrast agents may not be widely available at most institutions. Moreover, CE-IOUS requires a skilled operator to navigate the equipment and interpret the images in real time. Systemic adoption of CE-IOUS and ultimate widespread use will require significant investment on the part of individual surgeons, care teams, and hospital systems.

SUMMARY

CE-IOUS is a relatively new adjunct tool that allows for real-time contrast-enhanced imaging of the liver. In patients with cirrhotic livers, CE-IOUS can help characterize indeterminate lesions detected on conventional IOUS and distinguish HCC from dysplastic or regenerative nodules. For patients with CRLM, CE-IOUS can more sensitively detect small sites of liver metastases that may not be apparent on previous imaging. Ultimately, new information yielded using CE-IOUS can influence surgical decision-making and may contribute to improved outcomes for patients undergoing surgery for HCC or CRLM.

CLINICS CARE POINTS

- CE-IOUS uses pure blood pool contrast agents that are safe and provide real-time dynamic enhancement patterns of liver. The acquisition of the appropriate ultrasound equipment, contrast-specific software, UCA, and adequate practitioner training in both performing CE-IOUS and interpreting images are required to perform CE-IOUS.

- CE-IOUS can increase the accurate detection of HCC nodules in patients with liver cirrhosis with sensitivities of 65% to 100% and specificities of 83% to 100%.[19,23–25] New information yielded by CE-IOUS can affect surgical decision-making with reports of 25% to 35% of patients undergoing modified operative decisions as a result of CE-IOUS findings.[19]

- For patients with known or suspected CRLM, CE-IOUS is a valuable tool that can improve the sensitive detection of metastases. Although Gd-EOB-MRI has demonstrated benefit over CE-CT for the detection of small liver metastases, CE-IOUS may still be a useful adjunct modality with studies demonstrating improved sensitivity of detection of DLMs from 48% to 93% in patients with CRLM with the sequential use of Gd-EOB-MRI and CE-IOUS.[40,41]

DISCLOSURE

The authors have nothing to disclose.

REFERENCES

1. Makuuchi M, Hasegawa H, Yamazaki S. Ultrasonically guided subsegmentectomy. Surg Gynecol Obstet 1985;161(4):346–50.
2. Rifkin MD, Rosato FE, Branch HM, et al. Intraoperative ultrasound of the liver. An important adjunctive tool for decision making in the operating room. Ann Surg 1987;205(5):466–72.
3. Durot I, Wilson SR, Willmann JK. Contrast-enhanced ultrasound of malignant liver lesions. Abdom Radiol (NY) 2018;43(4):819–47.

4. Malone CD, Fetzer DT, Monsky WL, et al. Contrast-enhanced US for the interventional radiologist: current and emerging applications. Radiographics 2020;40(2): 562–88.

5. Torzilli G, Del Fabbro D, Olivari N, et al. Contrast-enhanced ultrasonography during liver surgery. Br J Surg 2004;91(9):1165–7.

6. Ranganath PG, Robbin ML, Back SJ, et al. Practical advantages of contrast-enhanced ultrasound in abdominopelvic radiology. Abdom Radiol (NY) 2018; 43(4):998–1012.

7. Barr RG. How to develop a contrast-enhanced ultrasound program. J Ultrasound Med 2017;36(6):1225–40.

8. Maruyama H, Sekimoto T, Yokosuka O. Role of contrast-enhanced ultrasonography with Sonazoid for hepatocellular carcinoma: evidence from a 10-year experience. J Gastroenterol 2016;51(5):421–33.

9. Yanagisawa K, Moriyasu F, Miyahara T, et al. Phagocytosis of ultrasound contrast agent microbubbles by Kupffer cells. Ultrasound Med Biol 2007;33(2):318–25.

10. Claudon M, Dietrich CF, Choi BI, et al. Guidelines and good clinical practice recommendations for contrast enhanced ultrasound (CEUS) in the liver–update 2012: a WFUMB-EFSUMB initiative in cooperation with representatives of AFSUMB, AIUM, ASUM, FLAUS and ICUS. Ultraschall Med 2013;34(1):11–29.

11. Dietrich CF, Averkiou M, Nielsen MB, et al. How to perform Contrast-Enhanced Ultrasound (CEUS). Ultrasound Int Open 2018;4(1):E2–15.

12. Piscaglia F, Bolondi L. Italian Society for Ultrasound in Medicine and Biology (SIUMB) Study Group on ultrasound contrast agents. The safety of Sonovue in abdominal applications: retrospective analysis of 23188 investigations. Ultrasound Med Biol 2006;32(9):1369–75.

13. An efficacy and safety study of Sonazoid and SonoVue in participants with focal liver lesions, undergoing pre- and post-contrast ultrasound imaging. ClinicalTrials.gov identifier: NCT03335566. Available at: https://clinicaltrials.gov/ct2/show/NCT03335566. Accessed December 20, 2021.

14. Lv K, Zhai H, Jiang Y, et al. Prospective assessment of diagnostic efficacy and safety of SonazoidTM and SonoVue® ultrasound contrast agents in patients with focal liver lesions. Abdom Radiol (NY) 2021;46(10):4647–59.

15. Kim TK, Noh SY, Wilson SR, et al. Contrast-enhanced ultrasound (CEUS) liver imaging reporting and data system (LI-RADS) 2017 - a review of important differences compared to the CT/MRI system. Clin Mol Hepatol 2017;23(4):280–9.

16. American College of Radiology Committee on LI-RADS® (Liver). CEUS LI-RADS® v2017 CORE. Available at: https://www.acr.org/Clinical-Resources/Reporting-and-Data-Systems/LI-RADS/CEUS-LI-RADS-v2017.   American College of Radiology. Accessed on December 21, 2021.

17. Donadon M, Torzilli G. Intraoperative ultrasound in patients with hepatocellular carcinoma: from daily practice to future trends. Liver Cancer 2013;2(1):16–24.

18. Zhang K, Kokudo N, Hasegawa K, et al. Detection of new tumors by intraoperative ultrasonography during repeated hepatic resections for hepatocellular carcinoma. Arch Surg 2007;142(12):1170–6.

19. Torzilli G, Palmisano A, Del Fabbro D, et al. Contrast-enhanced intraoperative ultrasonography during surgery for hepatocellular carcinoma in liver cirrhosis: is it useful or useless? A prospective cohort study of our experience. Ann Surg Oncol 2007;14(4):1347–55.

20. Takigawa Y, Sugawara Y, Yamamoto J, et al. New lesions detected by intraoperative ultrasound during liver resection for hepatocellular carcinoma. Ultrasound Med Biol 2001;27(2):151–6.

21. Torzilli G, Minagawa M, Takayama T, et al. Accurate preoperative evaluation of liver mass lesions without fine-needle biopsy. Hepatology 1999;30(4):889–93.
22. Joo I. The role of intraoperative ultrasonography in the diagnosis and management of focal hepatic lesions. Ultrasonography 2015;34(4):246–57.
23. Arita J, Takahashi M, Hata S, et al. Usefulness of contrast-enhanced intraoperative ultrasound using Sonazoid in patients with hepatocellular carcinoma. Ann Surg 2011;254(6):992–9.
24. Mitsunori Y, Tanaka S, Nakamura N, et al. Contrast-enhanced intraoperative ultrasound for hepatocellular carcinoma: high sensitivity of diagnosis and therapeutic impact. J Hepatobiliary Pancreat Sci 2013;20(2):234–42.
25. Abo T, Nanashima A, Tobinaga S, et al. Usefulness of intraoperative diagnosis of hepatic tumors located at the liver surface and hepatic segmental visualization using indocyanine green-photodynamic eye imaging. Eur J Surg Oncol 2015; 41(2):257–64.
26. Zhai HY, Liang P, Yu J, et al. Comparison of sonazoid and sonovue in the diagnosis of focal liver lesions: a preliminary study. J Ultrasound Med 2019;38(9): 2417–25.
27. Engstrand J, Nilsson H, Strömberg C, et al. Colorectal cancer liver metastases - a population-based study on incidence, management and survival. BMC Cancer 2018;18(1):78.
28. Evrard S, Poston G, Kissmeyer-Nielsen P, et al. Combined ablation and resection (CARe) as an effective parenchymal sparing treatment for extensive colorectal liver metastases. PLoS One 2014;9(12):e114404.
29. Imai K, Allard MA, Benitez CC, et al. Early recurrence after hepatectomy for colorectal liver metastases: what optimal definition and what predictive factors? Oncologist 2016;21(7):887–94.
30. Fergadi MP, Magouliotis DE, Vlychou M, et al. A meta-analysis evaluating contrast-enhanced intraoperative ultrasound (CE-IOUS) in the context of surgery for colorectal liver metastases. Abdom Radiol (NY) 2021;46(9):4178–88.
31. Liu W, Zhang ZY, Yin SS, et al. Contrast-enhanced intraoperative ultrasound improved sensitivity and positive predictive value in colorectal liver metastasis: a systematic review and meta-analysis. Ann Surg Oncol 2021;28(7):3763–73.
32. Stavrou GA, Stang A, Raptis DA, et al. Intraoperative (Contrast-Enhanced) ultrasound has the highest diagnostic accuracy of any imaging modality in resection of colorectal liver metastases. J Gastrointest Surg 2021;25(12):3160–9.
33. Benoist S, Brouquet A, Penna C, et al. Complete response of colorectal liver metastases after chemotherapy: does it mean cure? J Clin Oncol 2006;24(24): 3939–45.
34. Muaddi H, Silva S, Choi WJ, et al. When is a ghost really gone? A systematic review and meta-analysis of the accuracy of imaging modalities to predict complete pathological response of colorectal cancer liver metastases after chemotherapy. Ann Surg Oncol 2021;28(11):6805–13.
35. Shiozawa K, Watanabe M, Ikehara T, et al. Comparison of contrast-enhanced ultrasonograpy with Gd-EOB-DTPA-enhanced MRI in the diagnosis of liver metastasis from colorectal cancer. J Clin Ultrasound 2017;45(3):138–44.
36. Hatanaka K, Kudo M, Minami Y, et al. Sonazoid-enhanced ultrasonography for diagnosis of hepatic malignancies: comparison with contrast-enhanced CT. Oncology 2008;75(Suppl 1):42–7.
37. Hammerstingl R, Huppertz A, Breuer J, et al. Diagnostic efficacy of gadoxetic acid (Primovist)-enhanced MRI and spiral CT for a therapeutic strategy:

comparison with intraoperative and histopathologic findings in focal liver lesions. Eur Radiol 2008;18(3):457–67.

38. Muhi A, Ichikawa T, Motosugi U, et al. Diagnosis of colorectal hepatic metastases: comparison of contrast-enhanced CT, contrast-enhanced US, superparamagnetic iron oxide-enhanced MRI, and gadoxetic acid-enhanced MRI. J Magn Reson Imaging 2011;34(2):326–35.

39. Iwamoto T, Imai Y, Kogita S, et al. Comparison of contrast-enhanced ultrasound and gadolinium-ethoxybenzyl-diethylenetriamine pentaacetic acid-enhanced MRI for the diagnosis of macroscopic type of hepatocellular carcinoma. Dig Dis 2016;34(6):679–86.

40. Oba A, Mise Y, Ito H, et al. Clinical implications of disappearing colorectal liver metastases have changed in the era of hepatocyte-specific MRI and contrast-enhanced intraoperative ultrasonography. HPB (Oxford) 2018;20(8):708–14.

41. Arita J, Ono Y, Takahashi M, et al. Routine preoperative liver-specific magnetic resonance imaging does not exclude the necessity of contrast-enhanced intraoperative ultrasound in hepatic resection for colorectal liver metastasis. Ann Surg 2015;262(6):1086–91.

UNITED STATES POSTAL SERVICE® Statement of Ownership, Management, and Circulation (All Periodicals Publications Except Requester Publications)

1. Publication Title	2. Publication Number	3. Filing Date
SURGICAL ONCOLOGY CLINICS OF NORTH AMERICA	012 – 565	9/18/2022

4. Issue Frequency	5. Number of Issues Published Annually	6. Annual Subscription Price
JAN, APR, JUL, OCT	4	$325.00

7. Complete Mailing Address of Known Office of Publication (Not printer) (Street, city, county, state, and ZIP+4®)

ELSEVIER INC.
230 Park Avenue, Suite 800
New York, NY 10169

Contact Person
Malathi Samayan

Telephone (Include area code)
91-44-4299-4507

8. Complete Mailing Address of Headquarters or General Business Office of Publisher (Not printer)

ELSEVIER INC.
230 Park Avenue, Suite 800
New York, NY 10169

9. Full Names and Complete Mailing Addresses of Publisher, Editor, and Managing Editor (Do not leave blank)

Publisher (Name and complete mailing address)

Dolores Meloni, ELSEVIER INC.
1600 JOHN F KENNEDY BLVD. SUITE 1800
PHILADELPHIA, PA 19103-2899

Editor (Name and complete mailing address)

JOHN VASSALLO, ELSEVIER INC.
1600 JOHN F KENNEDY BLVD. SUITE 1800
PHILADELPHIA, PA 19103-2899

Managing Editor (Name and complete mailing address)

PATRICK MANLEY, ELSEVIER INC.
1600 JOHN F KENNEDY BLVD. SUITE 1800
PHILADELPHIA, PA 19103-2899

10. Owner (Do not leave blank. If the publication is owned by a corporation, give the name and address of the corporation immediately followed by the names and addresses of all stockholders owning or holding 1 percent or more of the total amount of stock. If not owned by a corporation, give the names and addresses of the individual owners. If owned by a partnership or other unincorporated firm, give its name and address as well as those of each individual owner. If the publication is published by a nonprofit organization, give its name and address.)

Full Name	Complete Mailing Address
WHOLLY OWNED SUBSIDIARY OF REED/ELSEVIER, US HOLDINGS	1600 JOHN F KENNEDY BLVD. SUITE 1800 PHILADELPHIA, PA 19103-2899

11. Known Bondholders, Mortgagees, and Other Security Holders Owning or Holding 1 Percent or More of Total Amount of Bonds, Mortgages, or Other Securities. If none, check box → ☐ None

Full Name	Complete Mailing Address
N/A	

12. Tax Status (For completion by nonprofit organizations authorized to mail at nonprofit rates) (Check one)
The purpose, function, and nonprofit status of this organization and the exempt status for federal income tax purposes:
☒ Has Not Changed During Preceding 12 Months
☐ Has Changed During Preceding 12 Months (Publisher must submit explanation of change with this statement)

PS Form 3526, July 2014 [Page 1 of 4 (see instructions page 4)]   PSN: 7530-01-000-9931   PRIVACY NOTICE: See our privacy policy on www.usps.com.

---

13. Publication Title		14. Issue Date for Circulation Data Below
SURGICAL ONCOLOGY CLINICS OF NORTH AMERICA		JULY 2022

15. Extent and Nature of Circulation			Average No. Copies Each Issue During Preceding 12 Months	No. Copies of Single Issue Published Nearest to Filing Date
a. Total Number of Copies (Net press run)			102	98
b. Paid Circulation (By Mail and Outside the Mail)	(1)	Mailed Outside-County Paid Subscriptions Stated on PS Form 3541 (Include paid distribution above nominal rate, advertiser's proof copies, and exchange copies)	41	36
	(2)	Mailed In-County Paid Subscriptions Stated on PS Form 3541 (Include paid distribution above nominal rate, advertiser's proof copies, and exchange copies)	0	0
	(3)	Paid Distribution Outside the Mails Including Sales Through Dealers and Carriers, Street Vendors, Counter Sales, and Other Paid Distribution Outside USPS®	32	34
	(4)	Paid Distribution by Other Classes of Mail Through the USPS (e.g., First-Class Mail®)	0	0
c. Total Paid Distribution (Sum of 15b (1), (2), (3), and (4))			73	70
d. Free or Nominal Rate Distribution (By Mail and Outside the Mail)	(1)	Free or Nominal Rate Outside-County Copies included on PS Form 3541	13	11
	(2)	Free or Nominal Rate In-County Copies Included on PS Form 3541	0	0
	(3)	Free or Nominal Rate Copies Mailed at Other Classes Through the USPS (e.g., First-Class Mail)	0	0
	(4)	Free or Nominal Rate Distribution Outside the Mail (Carriers or other means)	0	0
e. Total Free or Nominal Rate Distribution (Sum of 15d (1), (2), (3) and (4))			13	11
f. Total Distribution (Sum of 15c and 15e)			86	81
g. Copies not Distributed (See Instructions to Publishers #4 (page #3))			16	17
h. Total (Sum of 15f and g)			102	98
i. Percent Paid (15c divided by 15f times 100)			84.88%	86.41%

* If you are claiming electronic copies, go to line 16 on page 3. If you are not claiming electronic copies, skip to line 17 on page 3.

16. Electronic Copy Circulation		Average No. Copies Each Issue During Preceding 12 Months	No. Copies of Single Issue Published Nearest to Filing Date
a. Paid Electronic Copies	▲		
b. Total Paid Print Copies (Line 15c) + Paid Electronic Copies (Line 16a)	▲		
c. Total Print Distribution (Line 15f) + Paid Electronic Copies (Line 16a)	▲		
d. Percent Paid (Both Print & Electronic Copies) (16b divided by 16c × 100)	▲		

☒ I certify that 50% of all my distributed copies (electronic and print) are paid above a nominal price.

17. Publication of Statement of Ownership

☒ If the publication is a general publication, publication of this statement is required. Will be printed   ☐ Publication not required.
in the   OCTOBER 2022   issue of this publication.

18. Signature and Title of Editor, Publisher, Business Manager, or Owner

Malathi Samayan   Malathi Samayan - Distribution Controller   Date   9/18/2022

I certify that all information furnished on this form is true and complete. I understand that anyone who furnishes false or misleading information on this form or who omits material or information requested on the form may be subject to criminal sanctions (including fines and imprisonment) and/or civil sanctions (including civil penalties).

PS Form 3526, July 2014 (Page 2 of 4)   PRIVACY NOTICE: See our privacy policy on www.usps.com

Printed and bound by CPI Group (UK) Ltd, Croydon, CR0 4YY

03/10/2024

01040476-0013